Andrew Stanway

Alternative Medicine

A Guide to Natural Therapies

Penguin Books

Penguin Books Ltd, Harmondsworth, Middlesex, England
Viking Penguin Inc., 40 West 23rd Street, New York, New York 10010, U.S.A.
Penguin Books Australia Ltd, Ringwood, Victoria, Australia
Penguin Books Canada Limited, 2801 John Street, Markham, Ontario, Canada L3R 1B4
Penguin Books (N.Z.) Ltd, 182–190 Wairau Road, Auckland 10, New Zealand

First published in Great Britain by Macdonald and Jane's 1980
Published in Penguin Books in the United States
of America by arrangement with The
Rainbird Publishing Group Ltd, 40 Park Street,
London W1Y 4DE
Published in Pelican Books 1982
Reprinted with revisions in Penguin Books 1986

Filmset, printed and bound in Great Britain by
Hazell Watson & Viney Limited, Aylesbury, Bucks
Member of the BPCC Group
Set in VIP Times

Penguin Health
Alternative Medicine

Dr Andrew Stanway, MB, MRCP, practised medicine on the
Professorial Medical Unit at King's Hospital in London
before leaving to edit medical journals for doctors for five
years. In 1973 he started a medical film company, making
educational and documentary films for doctors, dentists,
health-care professionals and TV around the world. He has
written seventeen books, including *A Dictionary of
Operations*, *Taking the Rough with the Smooth*, *The Boots
Book of First Aid*, *Overcoming Depression*, *Why Us? – A
Guide for Infertile Couples*, *Alternative Medicine: A Guide to
Natural Therapies*, and four titles with his wife, Dr Penny
Stanway, about family life, including *Breast is Best*, an
international bestseller about breastfeeding, *The Baby and
Child Book* and *The Complete Book of Love and Sex: A
Guide for All The Family*, with Dr Philip Cauthery. He is also
co-author, with Dr Philip Cauthery and Faye Cooper, of *The
Complete Guide to Sexual Fulfilment*. His books on
depression and infertility took him further into the area of
sexual problems and their effects on people's lives, and he
has since become increasingly active clinically in this field.

Dr Stanway has been interested in alternative medicine for
ten years and is very active in promoting it. He was a
Founder Trustee of the Institute for Complementary
Medicine in London, an organization devoted to encouraging
the future of alternative medicine by fostering research,
coordinating political activities, widening public
understanding and offering a free information service
nationwide.

Since then he has been involved in numerous educational
and commercial projects in the natural health arena. He is
editor of the book *Natural Family Doctor* and technical
adviser to a major international TV series about alternative
medicine.

Contents

6 *Alternative Medicine*

Foreword

In 1961 I was asked to find out how the therapies mentioned in a book called *The Pattern of Health* by Dr Aubrey Westlake worked. Aubrey is a physician who has been researching and practising alternative therapies for over fifty years and old enough to be my father. I went to see him with an open mind, but at that time I was an orthodox medical practitioner who was both ignorant and sceptical of 'all this quackery'. We got on together well. He showed me cancer sufferers who, but for his 'quackery', ought to have died long ago. In the course of many long conversations he explained his views on how the natural therapies worked. Consequently, though it was at that time frowned upon by the General Medical Council in Britain, I began telling those patients whom I could not help with orthodox medicine to consult practitioners of other systems. There were many successes. I also began to use the Bach flower remedies in my private practice, swearing patients to secrecy. As a result, although I was only a general physician, I began to acquire a reputation as a psychotherapist. Eventually I was asked to join the Healing Research Trust and wrote a book on Natural Therapies called *Try Being Healthy*, giving my experience over fifteen years.

It was a pleasant surprise to be consulted by Dr Andrew Stanway before he started writing this book. Andrew gave up medicine in favour of writing and film making when he was a medical registrar and on the way to being a medical specialist, so he brings a critical and well-informed mind to the subject. Not only that, but his years of experience as a medical journalist, an editor and author, plus a natural talent, have led to him having an unusually lucid and easily read style. This is a real advantage in a field where medical practitioners and natural therapists writing about their subjects tend to be tortuous and polysyllabic. It ensures that the book will serve as a guide not only to the public which wants to know more about the natural therapies, but also as an introduction to the subject for the medical profession, especially now that doctors are increasingly referring their patients to practitioners of the natural therapies.

Andrew is young enough to be my son. He too was open-minded when he first came to see me. It is clear that a thorough examination of the subject has led him to the conclusion that many natural therapies work. As the go-between, I would like to congratulate Drs Andrew Stanway and Aubrey Westlake as the author and grandfather respectively of *Alternative Medicine: a Guide to Natural Therapies*.

This is a splendid book. I am sure that it will have the success that such clear and sensible writing on an important subject deserves.

Alec Forbes, MA, DM(Oxon), FRCP
Plymouth

Preface

Writing a book about alternative medical therapies is no easy matter. For a start there are so many of them. The Medical Faculty of the University of Rome convened the first World Congress on Alternative Medicine in 1973 and the provisional programme contained no less than 135 different therapies. Clearly, a book of this size could not cover all of these, so I have concentrated on those topics that either have a distinguished past, a promising present or future or are simply fascinating in their own right. I really see little use for urine therapy and the chances that gem therapy will ever be a meaningful part of western health care are small! In making this selection I hope I have not missed out anything important but would be pleased to hear from any reader who thinks I have.

Only a couple of centuries ago medicine was a blend of art, science, myth, magic and superstition. Today it is overwhelmingly a scientific extension of twentieth-century technology and the other facets have become either unacceptable or have been so ridiculed as to render them worthless. We are currently experiencing a widening of horizons and a breaking down of barriers in the West. Meditation, ways of controlling the mind, oriental religions, a greater interest in healthy eating, greater awareness of the problems of pollution and a growing sense of Man as a part of a larger world are all enjoying a wide public following. In spite of a general movement towards naturalness which is touching families who would by no means align themselves with the way-out fringes, the western medical profession continues to plod the never ending and increasingly frustrating path of orthodox health care.

Orthodox medicine has little time for the fringe – and vice versa. The orthodox fear the very real dangers associated with an upsurge of quacks and charlatans taking people's money and promising them the earth. The fringe fear that modern orthodox medicine is too bigoted and blinkered to be able to recognize a useful fringe therapy if it saw it and altogether the atmosphere is an unhappy one. There is no need for this. Orthodox medicine has its place and none of the alternatives can answer all of the world's health problems on its own. Most, but especially those such as colour therapy and the Alexander technique, are not pretending to be total health care systems anyway but simply auxiliaries to existing medical care.

As a qualified doctor I have tried to look at these therapies in a rather new light. Other books have been written about alternative therapies but almost without exception they are written by the therapists themselves. This has its disadvantages – not the least of which is that many of them are so close to their subjects that, with a few notable exceptions, they can't stand back and take a detached view. This leads to an inbreeding I see all too often in orthodox medical circles and also breeds the same kinds of petty bickering one sees among scientific ultra experts who can only really communicate with a handful of people on their level.

In writing the book I have taken great pains to see either the person who invented the therapy or his co-workers or successors. In this way I hope that I've been able to present a picture as close as possible to the original. All successful human studies and endeavours evolve but often the evolution involves perversions and distortions of the original concept. By sticking closely to the originator's own work I hope to have overcome much of this problem.

Clearly as a doctor I cannot possibly recommend all these therapies. First of all, I simply haven't enough experience of most of them to be able to be sure and second, I would not be so rash as to recommend something for a patient (or reader) whom I had never met and assessed personally. However, by seeing medical practitioners who use these methods either full time or substantially part time I think I've been able to satisfy myself that each works for certain conditions. No *one* therapy claims to be able to cope with every disease and on average I find a far greater willingness to accept this among fringe practitioners than I do among orthodox practitioners.

Lastly, I make no apologies for the fact that I approach patients as people who are highly complex physical and spiritual creatures. Modern medical 'plumbing' has no attraction for me and I know from experience that I am not alone! Fifteen years listening to the public and writing for them have taught me that people want a medical care system that gets them better with the least possible intervention, be it from investigations, drugs or operations. The very nature of a medical care system that treats all patients with the same disease label as though they were the same person militates against the individual treatment that people so enjoy and look for in their medical care. The modern medical conveyor belt often loses sight of people as individuals – much to the chagrin of patient and doctor alike.

The alternative medical therapies I've covered in this book deserve serious consideration by the medical and scientific communities. Alas, their very nature often renders this difficult and, because it is so difficult, many people are all too ready to condemn them. My researches show that most of these therapies have far more to recommend them than most people realize and that they urgently deserve more research and attention. Such a move is unlikely to come from within the medical profession – so it's up to you!

Andrew Stanway

Acknowledgements

I should like to thank the following practitioners whose help has been invaluable in writing this book:
Dr Wilfred Barlow, Mr R. Bloomfield, Dr L. Charles, Mrs Kay Corden, Mr T. G. Dummer, Dr J. Dyson, Mr M. Endacott, Mr Theo Gimbel, Mrs G. Hemmings, Dr E. Holiday, Mr I. M. Hutchinson, Dr C. O. Kennedy, Mr D. J. Kieley, Mr C. A. Laws, Dr Felix Mann, Mr P. G. Manners, Lt Col. M. McCausland, Malcolm Rae, Danièle Ryman, Mr Ian Scott, Mr R. A. Stenstadvold, Bill Tara, Mr R. B. Tisserand, Mr G. Tridgell, Mrs A. Warren-Davis, Dr A. T. Westlake, Dr A. Woolley-Hart.

My special thanks are due to Dr Alec Forbes, Senior Consultant Physician at a large hospital, for writing the Foreword and for his help and guidance throughout.

Illustration Acknowledgements

The publishers would like to thank Marion Appleton for the illustrations on pp. 21, 70–71, 84–6, 142–3, 144, 178–9, 181, 255, 290, 291 and the Unit for the Study of Health Policy, Department of Community Medicine, Guy's Hospital Medical School, for their help.

Introduction

Before looking at the different types of alternative medicine and at what each has to offer, it is helpful to look at the present pattern of medical care available in the West. After all, alternative medicine is, by definition, an alternative to something else. That 'something else' is modern, western medicine. But before we go any further, it's important to understand that this book is not about *the* alternative to orthodox medicine – simply *an* alternative or, more accurately, many alternatives. The concept of an alternative is a relative one and public and medical opinions are changing all the time. Yesterday's alternative can be part of today's orthodox. It might be better, then, to consider the therapies covered in this book as *supplements* to orthodox medicine, because, as we shall see, I have nowhere suggested that they should take over *instead of* western medicine.

Recently the word 'complementary' has been applied to many of these therapies. The dictionary defines a complement as 'something that serves to make whole', and many such therapies could be thought of in these terms. Those who favour the word claim that the therapies bring an individual back to wholeness and so are worthy of the name. Most people, however, think that the word complementary means that both types of therapy should be used side by side so that the consumer gets the best of both worlds. In principle this is fine, but in practice it isn't so easy, because the vast majority of orthodox practitioners certainly don't think of the therapies discussed in this book as complementary to their practice. Because the so-called complementary therapies usually call for a rather different view of health, illness and cure from that used by orthodox practitioners, they are often at loggerheads on the very basics of the therapies.

So it is that a doctor thinks he can learn herbal medicine in a weekend or become an acupuncturist after a short course. Neither, of course, is possible, because both require a considerable leap in thinking about health and disease as the ground rules are very different in such natural therapies. Most doctors think they can take the best of the alternative therapies and add them on to their existing practices, rather as if they had acquired a new medical gadget, whereas the natural therapist sees this as yet another gimmick as orthodox medics try to jump on the bandwagon of 'naturalness'.

For these and many other reasons I see the natural therapies as being 'alternative' for a very long time to come. Current medical thinking along Cartesian lines has taken hundreds of years to evolve and there is no real sign that doctors will do anything more than pick and choose at the most superficial applications of some of the better known therapies. There is no evidence that the changes of philosophy so urgently required, and which are so in line with the natural therapies, are occurring on any significant scale.

The way out of the dilemma is, in my view, to call the therapies in this book 'natural' therapies. This doesn't mean that western medicine is *un*natural but that many, if not most, of those so often called 'alternative' work on the basis of nature providing the cure – with human beings to help it along. Just because something is 'natural' doesn't, of course, make it better, but in the context of natural therapies this turns out to be the case very often. Given that so many conditions are self-limiting, as we shall see, all that is required is that the body be given the 'raw materials' to heal itself. Often, western medicine seems to do exactly the reverse.

People have always wanted alternative forms of medical therapy to those which are readily available, but today in the West the need is apparently greater than ever. This has probably come about for five main reasons: people see orthodox therapies failing in certain conditions (especially chronic ones) and find this hard to accept; many are afraid of western medical treatment with its operations and drug side-effects; some people have religious or philosophical arguments against certain western medical practices; there is a growing minority of people of all ages which feels it is time to protest about what *is* available; and lastly there always has been and hopefully always will be a proportion of the population which simply needs to be different and to experiment, and this extends to the kinds of medical care it demands. But whatever the reason for choosing alternative or orthodox therapies, the starting point is the same – an ill person.

A substantial proportion of people does nothing at all for minor aches, pains and everyday ailments, yet they improve. This is a fact to bear in mind from the start: there are large numbers of complaints that get better by themselves whatever action the sufferer takes. There is, of course, a step between doing nothing at all and seeking outside help, and that is to cure oneself. Millions of people the world over are doing just this every day: granny's cures for colds and 'flu abound and each nation and even region within a nation develops its own remedies for common ailments. 'Self-medication' is encouraged by pharmaceutical and other companies and all over the world there are patent medicines available which promise great things in return for a small outlay. Apart from this similarity to other parts of the world, however, medicine is very different in the West, where healing is dominated by technological medicine and where the orthodox medical profession has helped to make any other type of healing illegal or socially unacceptable. There are some encouraging signs that things are changing, as we shall see on page 35.

When someone seeks medical help they are usually suffering from one of four groups of conditions. The condition may be self-limiting as we've already seen; it may be chronic, with an uneven succession of partial recoveries and relapses (the 'It's my old trouble again, doctor' story); it may be of psychological origin (caused by difficulties with family and interpersonal relationships, work trouble, poor housing, money problems and so on); or it might actually be an acute medical condition.

All of these people really *are* ill and will benefit from some sort of treatment. Those with a self-limiting illness would have got better anyway; the chronically ill can be offered symptomatic relief but know that their condition fluctuates and that their improvement might not have been brought about by the treatment; the psychologically-based group needs understanding and help (much of which need not necessarily, or even ideally, come from a doctor) and the last group gets most benefit from modern western medicine.

The trouble with most people in the western world is that they imagine that doctors spend their time seeing and curing this last group. In reality this group makes up less than 20 per cent of those going to doctors. The other 80 per cent fall into the other three groups and simply don't *need* western medicine *per se*. Many of them would fare just as well if they didn't live in the sophisticated western world, and from a sociological standpoint many would fare better in a society in which family ties were stronger and a sense of close community help more meaningful than it is in the West today.

There is also a widely held view that medical advances in the western world enable us to live longer. This is not necessarily true. The search for a cure for all our ills and for ways of prolonging life has exercised human minds for centuries. Indeed, it was the inability to accept these ills as inevitable which first led to human interest in medicine as a discipline.

In the past, war, famine and pestilence ensured that of those who survived the childhood infections, few survived adulthood and even fewer reached old age. A baby born at the time of the Emperor Augustus could only expect to live for twenty-three years, according to a paper in the *Medical Journal of Australia* in 1964. It says, 'there was almost certainly no gain during the Middle Ages, but life expectancy slowly increased during modern times and by 1850 had reached forty years. By 1900 another upward move had brought it up to forty-seven years.

Today, in most western countries, life expectancy at birth has reached the impressive figure of seventy years.' But the author then goes on to warn, 'Our smug satisfaction with the achievement, however, needs correction. While in the last century medical science succeeded in pushing life expectancy at birth up by some twenty years, the life expectancy of a sixty-five-year-old during the same period had risen by less than one year. To put it bluntly, while we have almost eradicated infectious illnesses of childhood and adulthood, we have not succeeded in preventing degenerative processes and malignant growth, the two most common diseases of middle life and old age.'

This sobering view is not individually held nor is it even an extreme one. As long ago as the seventeenth century, Edmund Halley, the English astronomer, created the first life tables. He found that the expectation of life for a sixty-year old in 1687 was 12·09 years. Two hundred years later a sixty-year-old had 12·2 years on average to live and by 1950 this had risen to only 15·7. So 263 years after the first surveys, a sixty-year-old individual was living just three and a half years longer! A triumph of modern medicine? I think not.

We have to face up to the fact that modern medicine as we know it has done little to cure or prevent disease when compared with the advantages conferred upon society by good sanitation, improved housing, smaller families and other social improvements.

The proof that this is so can be seen in almost any urban Medical Officer of Health's Annual Reports. In 1873 the Medical Officer of Health for the London suburb of Charlton wrote, 'Gentlemen, in my last annual summary I reported to you that the year 1872 was a particularly healthy year and the mortality exceptionally low and I am happy on the present occasion to state that, during the year 1873 the same high standard of health was continued. I cannot but attribute this diminished mortality which has now existed for some period . . . to the efficient inspection of the district by which all known nuisances or sources of disease are at once remedied or removed.' There were no cases of cholera that year and only four cases of typhoid. To put this into perspective, it was not uncommon for both these diseases to claim thousands of lives every year in the major cities of Britain until the middle of the nineteenth century.

What makes the impact of this Medical Officer's report all the more convincing is the fact that it was written more than ten years before medical science had even discovered that bacteria were the cause of cholera and typhoid – let alone come up with drugs to kill them.

Certainly, a handful of drug innovations has made a difference to life expectancy – for example, the antibiotics. But don't be fooled into thinking that they are responsible for saving as many millions of lives as you might think. After all, not everybody who suffered from even very severe infections died in the pre-antibiotic era, as any good physician or nurse of the day will confirm, and the majority of the killer infectious diseases was fast disappearing years before drugs were available to cure them! Even a killer condition such as tuberculosis, widely considered to have been wiped out by powerful antibiotics, was in fact eradicated not so much by these drugs as by improved social conditions. True, there *is* a handful of really useful drugs that has made meaningful inroads into disease and fatality figures but they are few indeed. Of far greater concern to many responsible doctors today are the millions of people being exposed to antibiotics (and to a certain extent this applies to other drugs too) unnecessarily. This over-exposure to drugs produces a whole new kind of illness, iatrogenic illness, disease actually brought about *by* doctors. Surveys that have tried to assess the amount of drug-induced illness are numerous and show that somewhere between 3 and 18 per cent of all patients in hospital are suffering from side-effects caused by their drug treatments. And this doesn't take into account the millions of people with side-effects from drugs who are going about their daily lives feeling 'not quit: right' yet not ill enough to go into hospital. There must be an alternative to this.

The price of modern medicine

So people are paying a heavy price for modern medicine and it's a price they may not have to pay. There is no one subject that disturbs people in the western health care system more than the seemingly massive overuse of drugs. The first movement away from what western medicine has to offer starts with a disenchantment or even a frank horror of what drugs do to people, mainly because going to the doctor has become synonymous with drug taking.

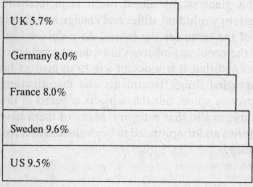

UK 5.7%

Germany 8.0%

France 8.0%

Sweden 9.6%

US 9.5%

Percentage of Gross National Product spent on health care in various countries in 1980
Source: OECD 1980

But the price we as a society pay for modern medicine is not only measured in unwanted drug side-effects and unnecessary investigations, but in money too. A recent survey in a British general practice illustrates this well. The doctors decided to stop prescribing drugs unless they were really necessary and started telling patients which conditions to bring to the doctor and which to treat themselves. In a single year they saved £20,000 which, taken for the country as a whole, would be a saving of £10m – just from this simple measure! But the illness business is vast and growing bigger daily as modern medicine gets more expensive and new gadgetry and equipment enable more sophisticated (and expensive) procedures to be carried out. In practice, modern medicine is becoming so expensive that it may soon have to be rationed simply because it will consume so enormous a part of any country's resources that the country won't be able to cope, and many sick people will go untreated.

Alternative medical methods, if widely implemented, could provide the answer to this problem. However, medicine is an enormous business and because big businesses are so well represented in high places, any change that is suggested is either squashed at once or ridiculed by the establishment as unworkable or useless. It is this giant establishment machine in medicine throughout the western world that stifles real change and simply encourages more of the same for the future. As a doctor I am only too aware of the problems inherent in frequent changes of ideas and therapies and that it is a doctor's duty to protect his patient from newfangled drugs, treatments and investigations until they are of proven value, but the subjects covered in this book are by and large not in that category. Many of them have been used for centuries and simply need to be evaluated in terms understandable today.

What is alternative medicine?

The term has come to embrace any form of medicine that is outside the main stream of western medicine as practised by the majority of doctors today. It is known as fringe medicine or more insultingly as 'quack' medicine because it is often practised by people with no formal medical training. In reality, of course, western medicine as we know it today is 'alternative medicine' in historic terms because many of the so-called fringe medical disciplines were going strong centuries or even thousands of years before modern medicine, which is only about 300 years old. Indeed, modern, drug-centred medicine is really only forty-five years old. Certainly, the ancients like Aristotle and Hippocrates and more recently Leonardo da Vinci made an enormous contribution to early medicine, but their impact on the health of the masses was tiny at the time. Until as recently as 150 years ago, plant extracts and simple inorganic compounds were the most useful treatments available, and it wasn't until the mid-1800s and the Listerian age of antiseptic surgery that safe, surgical techniques became anything like widespread. Certainly, we seem to have come a long way in the last century, but we haven't done much for our survival figures as we've already seen. We are simply dying of different things at much the same age. What modern medicine can do is cure some acute diseases and infections and relieve symptoms on a very wide scale. But in fairness we've also produced a large number of unpleasant side-effects from drugs, while operations like tonsillectomy, gall-bladder removal and appendectomy (to mention but a few) are often performed unnecessarily, creating needless suffering.

So before scoffing at alternative therapies, the modern doctor would do well to remember that very large numbers of the people who seek help with problems in the first three categories mentioned on page 17 would have been tolerably well treated even before the coming of modern medicine. And remember, this adds up to 80 per cent of those going to their doctors. Undoubtedly the other 20 per cent benefits from modern scientific medicine and I would be the last to put the clock back and allow my child or wife to die from appendicitis or any other acute, operable condition. However, not all surgery comes into the category of life-saving, modern medicine. The majority of surgery is done for hernias, varicose veins, piles and gall-stones – all to some extent preventable diseases. The amount of actual life-saving surgery carried out is tiny. Most surgeons are using space age technology to patch up our self-abused bodies and to make good the ravages of our modern nutrition and life style.

Modern medicine, then, is relatively new, much of it frankly untried for long enough and a lot of its efforts wasted (at great financial cost) simply because the sledgehammer is too big and the nut relatively small.

This will undoubtedly come as no surprise to readers, who will already have experienced as much in their own lives. But what can they do, living as they do within a modern monopoly health care situation? Very little, you may think, but you're wrong.

THERE'S NOTHING SACRED ABOUT WHAT MODERN MEDICINE HAS TO OFFER

We live in an age of consumerism and, by and large, that's no bad thing. The power in the hands of the man and woman in the street is enormous if they choose to wield it. I think this is what people should do all over the western world when it comes to alternative medicines. After all, all medical treatments are empirical – even (or especially, some cynics would say) 'technological' western medicine. If a treatment works, it works. It doesn't really matter what label it has on it. There's nothing sacred about what modern medicine has to offer – its benefits have often been achieved in other ways, frequently more cheaply and with fewer side-effects in the past or indeed somewhere today in another country. We tend to feel that because we in the West are the most industrially advanced we are somehow 'superior' to the millions in the developing countries of the world. Nothing could be further from the truth. A simple Buddhist monk may be a better, more successful, happier and more fulfilled person than many of us in the West, for all our medicine, washing machines and moon shots.

This brings me to an extremely important point in the introduction to alternative medicines – a brief discussion of the emphasis that western medicine puts on the mechanical side of the body, the 'plumbing'. All through medical school students learn of the arteries, the veins and the nerves of the body – where they are, how they work and what happens when they don't work. They are taught to discover what is wrong with a given part and then to attach a label to the malfunction. When – and only when – they have labelled something (this is called 'making a diagnosis') may they, or should they, treat it. This presents all thinking and honest doctors with an enormous dilemma, because they simply cannot adequately label so much of what they see and so feel inadequate themselves. Yet the importance of arriving at a diagnostic label has been so greatly stressed that they invariably do so, and when they do they diagnose a condition in terms of the 'plumbing' – because that's what they understand best.

But a person isn't a motor car – and is more than a collection of parts. In fact the more people know about the parts, the more questions they find. The notion, cherished by the popular press, that modern medicine is any nearer to understanding what humans are all about is completely false. Western and other therapists have huge and fundamental differences of opinion about the basic nature of the body. To many natural therapists the body's energy patterns are supremely important, yet orthodox physicians don't even admit that they exist. The functions of organs such as the liver are differently interpreted by many therapists and so on. We know a little about the plumbing, but by no means all there is to know. Only a few years ago a completely new nervous system was discovered – the VIPergic nervous system – that works by releasing vaso-active intestinal peptides. The trouble is that, with a few notable exceptions, most western doctors simply don't interest themselves in a lot of what natural therapists would call their 'plumbing', so modern medicine has hardly scratched the surface of what to the natural therapist are basic concerns. Kirlian photography is beginning to produce answers to this problem, but the results are patchy and vast amounts of money are needed to take this a step further so that diagnoses can be made from the body's 'subtle energies', as they are currently being made from electro-cardiograms, computerized tomography and magnetic resonance. Western technology is now in a position to really take the lid off human energy patterns and I hope that before long someone will start to do so. All of this still leaves a vast area that is badly taught, poorly understood and indeed almost ignored by modern western medicine – the mind, the soul and the spirit.

So badly have most doctors been trained in these areas that they can't even recognize a malfunction of the mind, soul or spirit when it stares them in the face – and even if they did, most of them wouldn't be adequately trained to cope with it. And all of this in the face of studies that have shown that up to 40 per cent of all patients seen by doctors in the West have nothing physically wrong with them at all. This emphasis on the plumbing to the almost total exclusion of other considerations has led to widespread distrust and disaffection and it is this as much as anything else that has made people turn to alternative therapies.

Most doctors become very angry when they hear this argument, but their anger is mostly protective, because they simply have not been taught to think on a plane other than a simple mechanical or biochemical one. At last a tiny ray of light is beginning to appear at the end of the tunnel and more doctors are becoming aware of phenomena such as psychogenic pain (pain brought on by psychological and not physical disease), psychosomatic illnesses (bodily disease manifestations of psychological disturbances), and spiritual suffering.

The supersensible world and a controlling force

In order to be able to grasp the significance of many of the alternative medical practices described in the book, readers will have to steer their minds on to rather a different plane from the one they are used to. As long as we continue to think of humans as a collection of working parts governed in the same way as a motor car, we'll have trouble understanding or even accepting many forms of natural medicine – simply because many of them work on the principle that people are not *only* highly sophisticated machines, but also have another, much more important, dimension.

There is an increasing awareness of another dimension of life that is not commonly experienced from day to day. Most of us have had telepathic experiences – husbands and wives often know exactly what the other is thinking and some people tell of how even their pets can read their thoughts. Many of us have met or heard of people who are psychic, or have been amazed by a clairvoyant, a fortune teller or other psychically active person. In fact, so widespread is the research into psychic matters, especially in the USSR, that it has become a branch of conventional science in its own right.

The problem most of us face when considering such paranormal phenomena is that we can't or won't accept that certain people might have something we haven't got or that they can perhaps tune in to another dimension of which we can't even conceive. This is simply human nature. We all like to think we're normal and that those who manifest special 'other worldly' skills are odd in some way. We tolerate them but are often a little alarmed, because they have an 'in' to a world we don't know about.

This all seems frightening to many of us and it was this kind of fear that led society to burn people as witches in the past. Today we are becoming more tolerant of such people and can actually see that they have things to teach us about the world in which we live.

Our world is presented to us through the inputs of our five physical senses. The output from these sophisticated and sensitive sense organs is interpreted by the brain and a balance of current and historic data (from our memories) gives us a fairly good idea of what's going on around us. Or so we think!

Actually, these interpretations are extremely limited – mainly because our sense organs, wonderful as they are, function only within very limited boundaries. For example, the human ear responds only to sounds within a frequency range of approximately 30–16,000 cycles per second. Animals and birds have hearing ranges which overlap the human range and some pick up high pitched sounds we can't hear. We all know about the 'silent' dog whistles that only dogs can hear and bats use even higher frequencies in their 'radar' systems. Some artificial inaudible vibrations are of an even higher frequency. It's apparent, then, that human ears pick up only a tiny fraction of everything there is to be 'heard'.

Our sense of sight is even more restricted. Our eyes respond to electromagnetic vibrations reflected off objects around us which make them perceivable by us. The spectrum of electromagnetic waves is vast, extending from certain intrinsic brain rhythms, through radio and TV waves to infra-red waves that we pick up as heat. There are about fifty octaves of electromagnetic radiations, yet our eyes pick up less than one! If our eyes could pick up even a few more frequencies – say the X-ray waves – then our whole perception of the outside world would be entirely different. The human sensory system seems to have been designed to enable us to cope adequately with our environment in biological terms. The fascinating thing is that of all these other 'potentially perceivable' vibrations around us, we only perceive a few. With vast areas of the brain not performing any function that we can measure (or appreciate, a lot of the time) it's highly likely that we could, under certain circumstances, extend our senses to take in some of these other 'vibrations'.

Unfortunately, all our ideas and concepts of life are restricted by our five physical senses. Yet the 'invisible' (for example, the minute structures that make up a human cell) is now visible using electron microscopes, while other equipment can pick up wave forms in the atmosphere of which we were ignorant until very recently. Our boundaries of perception are being extended all the time.

But in spite of this, we live in what the Hindus call Maya – an illusion. Our brains are tuned to select the available sensory stimuli in such a way that we are not aware of the inapparent yet nevertheless real world around us for the vast majority of our lives. Some people see more of this inapparent world than do the rest of us and certain people seem to be in touch with it a lot of the time.

In order really to understand the rest of our world we have to cast off our restrictive ways of thinking and envisage a *real* world larger than that which most of us appreciate with our five physical senses. This larger world (which I shall call the supersensible, or above the physical senses, world) can be appreciated by some of us by what is often called intuition, but this is probably simply a better developed ability to receive more of the available sensory stimuli. How many times have we had intuitive feelings about people, places, a new house, a second-hand car – the list is endless. The problem is that the only way that phenomena such as telepathy, clairvoyance and dowsing, for example, can be appreciated is by the mind and it's this that seems to be such a drawback to their acceptability in a technological age. Many of the available but inapparent stimuli around us are not measurable by methods currently used. However, modern techniques such as Kirlian photography are making headway here.

But just as our perceived surroundings are only a fraction of what there is to perceive, so it is with our bodies. Our physical bodies (which we can appreciate because our five physical senses tell us about them) are simply a part of a much larger whole. They (and indeed all living matter) generate and are subject to life forces – some of which are measurable. Many, however, are not perceivable through the five physical senses and can only be appreciated by the mind. On a day to day basis this restricted view of ourselves is all we need to be able to function adequately and our brains are not geared routinely to pick up people's body forces, TV, radio, radar and ultrasonic frequencies and feel colours. This is just as well, because we couldn't function as we do now in such a world. Many people – doctors, for example – use their 'sixth sense' many times a day and couldn't work effectively without doing so. In fact many of us often tune in to this higher, supersensible dimension without realizing it.

The great intuitive philosophers like Rudolf Steiner, the founder of anthroposophical medicine (see page 93), describe a higher body – the etheric body – which controls everything in the physical body. This is the same as the supersensible body I am describing and surrounds, influences and is influenced by our physical body. Unfortunately, even the term 'etheric' stirs up all that's most unreceptive in most of us, but this nineteenth-century, outmoded concept of the 'ether', whilst being outdated in simple terms, seems to make increasing sense scientifically.

The trouble is that we can only assess this etheric or supersensible world by inference – we have no ways of measuring it directly. We readily accept the concept of sub-atomic particles though we can't see them; we accept that people have intuitive feelings or knowledge of things, yet we can't measure intuition; so why can't we accept the existence of another 'higher', non-physical world more readily? I think it's for two reasons. First, many people have been conditioned to think of higher planes as being associated only with religion and there has been a decline in religion in the western world; and second, because we secretly fear things we can't measure or explain. Religion has a lot to answer for here and has been its own undoing in the West. Many religions start off promising an insight into and communication with this 'higher' world and can indeed give it. However, physical trappings often bog down higher intentions so that people either lose sight of the original purpose entirely or take a liking to the non-spiritual side of religion which then becomes an end in itself.

But just as we fear the possibility that there might be a whole world 'out there' that we can't readily perceive, we also hate to think that we might not be in control. We are in fact not in control in any real sense of anything at all – it's all part of the illusion of life. Take our bodies, for instance. Most of us assume that we're simply made up of cells built together in a cleverly structured way to form specific organs which keep us alive. What most people don't realize though is that the body is a constantly changing structure. Every second of our lives cells are dying and being replaced – in fact over a seven-year period most of our body structure will have been replaced. As we research deeper and deeper into cell structure we find that at the atomic level our whole body is simply a countless mass of energy fields all influencing each other. What we think of as solid tissue is in fact a mass of cells made up of families of chemical substances, in turn simply collections of atoms. Matter as such is a notional concept in terms of modern atomic physics. It's simply the result of atoms producing and reacting in energy fields. So as we look more deeply into the structure of human beings, we find that they can be reduced in physical terms to a collection of electromagnetic fields. What controls all these fields of energy at any one time? Science has no answers, but I maintain that the controlling forces are in the etheric or supersensible world we've been discussing. In other words, there come a point in our reductionist view of human beings when we can reduce no further, yet there is still a superior controlling force (that some call God) that seems to make it all work together harmoniously for most of the time. It is this superior controlling force that many alternative medical therapies harness to cure the patient. The sceptical scientist claims that eventually we'll be able to reduce the human body and indeed the universe to such a level that everything will be explicable in terms which our five physical senses can perceive, but there is no sign of this happening. On the contrary, the more we know, the more we realize how little we know and how immeasurably more complex everything is than we ever thought.

Once one accepts this supersensible world, it becomes apparent that events in life and bodily functions in particular are subject to two kinds of influence. There are the ordinary laws of cause and effect that influence all the world as we perceive it (if I cut myself, I bleed), and then there are other effects that arise from changes in the supersensible world – changes which transcend time and space. Every object in the real world also has a supersensible dimension but not all ailments, for example, are caused by supersensible changes. Some diseases arise from purely physical causes such as fractures or the blockage of a ureter by a kidney stone, and these can be made good by orthodox medical skills. In fact this is what orthodox medicine is best at doing.

The vast majority of illness though comes into a much broader category, as we have seen, and this bulk of ailments is probably the result of all kinds of disruptions, be they environmental, dietary, psychological or 'other worldly'. Once we bear in mind that the physical body is just a part of a much larger, if unmanifest, world that is directed by a superior power, we can better understand how it is that millions of people the world over have been practising forms of medicine entirely alien to us and our thinking quite successfully for thousands of years. The yogi who can alter the vital working of parts of his body (thought by medicine until recently to be completely uncontrollable) is only acceptable to us because we can measure these variables today, yet yogis have known for thousands of years that they could do it. The Ancients knew the importance of colour in healing yet it took the Russians to prove that humans can feel colour through the skin and that skin is infinitely more sensitive to sensations that ever we thought.

THE SOLELY INTELLECTUAL APPROACH TO SCIENCE GENERALLY AND MEDICINE IN PARTICULAR ISN'T PROVIDING THE ANSWERS

The beauty of all this is that we are all trainable. The vast majority of us has had paranormal experiences and can be trained by an expert to have many more.

This might seem unlikely to most readers but is in fact well within the realms of possibility. Matthew Manning, an exceptionally gifted psychic who is currently working with some of the world's leading academics in order to demonstrate and measure what is actually happening in various psychic phenomena, has described his work with a group of fifty people in Paris. The group had gathered to develop their psychic abilities. At the beginning of the two-day programme nobody could do anything, yet at the end 80 per cent were performing psychic functions as well as he could. It was simply because they knew *how* to do it, in what order to do things, how to visualize images. The only people it doesn't work for are people who have a conscious block. They say, 'These things don't happen to me' and prevent themselves doing them. Much of unorthodox medicine then simply works on a level we are untrained for. People are amazed at what they can achieve with a pendulum after a very short time (see page 268); the results of hypnosis astound others; yet others can't believe that their blood pressure can be raised by shining a red light on them; and others are astounded when they learn that they have healing powers in their hands. We're in for a great re-awakening of our non-physical senses in the next century, if only because we're realizing that the solely intellectual approach to science generally and medicine in particular isn't providing the answers. I hope we're coming out of the era of the 'intellectual individual' and entering a much higher plane of the 'supersensible individual'. This need not necessarily have anything to do with God or formalized religion as such; in fact some of the fringes of medicine or natural therapies seem to be contradictory to much of what formalized religion has to offer – at least in the West. It also has little to do with the spiritual or supernatural world as manifested by spiritualists. On the contrary, the abilities I am talking about are very much *of* humans. They are not *super*natural (above nature) – they are a part of nature. What many of the natural therapies demand is a basic humility – a willingness to accept that however much we know about the structure of the golf ball we will never be able to deduce from this alone the rules or attractions of golf as a game – and this humility is hard to find in our technological world.

Please don't let me give you the impression that I'm some sort of spiritualist quack or a doctor who thinks that patients 'imagine' their diseases. Far from it. But experience of nearly twenty years of talking to patients and doctors has taught me that we ignore the supersensible dimension of human beings at our peril, both within and outside medicine. However, millions of people actually believe that they are a glorified collection of car parts and expect that everything can be put right if only they can find a good enough mechanic. Alas, many people's experiences of western medicine are exactly analogous to the motor trade. They get their 'cars' back after two weeks with chipped parts badly fitted, giving problems they never had before and a bill for what they imagine must be a new car!

The search for the 'perfect mechanic', medically speaking, takes people from specialist to specialist in the hopes of finding answers to chronic diseases that no one can explain, let alone cure. All in all, we in western society are greatly over-doctored and interfered with and it is all of our own making. Today's family doctor is expected to be physician, marriage guidance expert, psychosexual counsellor, family therapist, teacher, priest and surrogate family member. Not surprisingly, doctors can't cope adequately with these demands, mainly because they have never been trained to do so, and give a less than good service in the areas where their competence *is* sound. This brings the technological wonders that they and western medicine can offer further into disrepute, and the extreme dependence of their patients upon them and the patients' implicit faith that they must have an answer to everything further demoralizes the doctor. I believe that it is for reasons such as these that natural medicine is now so popular with the public. Over the last twenty years or so people have become increasingly disenchanted with western, allopathic medicine, but the pace has hotted up over the last five years to the point where many westerners are now actually sceptical of it and unwilling to subject themselves and their families to it. In a recent study in Washington DC the majority of those asked to choose between a low-risk drug effective 50 per cent of the time, a high-risk (possibly carcinogenic) drug effective 100 per cent of the time, or a non-drug remedy that would help control the symptoms but not cure the problem, chose the last. For example, 81 per cent said they would rather go on a low-salt diet for their hypertension than take drugs.

The place of alternative therapies

This is where alternative medical therapies could play such an important role in the health care of the West. I do not wish to make a case for the abolition of western medicine. On the contrary, I'm suggesting that by taking advantage of the best alternative therapies and combining them with the finest in technological medicine, people would be able to enjoy a standard of health care that they have never yet seen – and at a much lower cost.

But for alternative therapies to be able to play their part in the total health care picture, a lot needs to happen.

First, doctors must be better trained to analyse and understand these therapies for what they are. Very few medical schools ever mention, for example, an ancient and valuable therapy such as herbal medicine, yet most of the world's medicines outside the West are what we would call herbal. By omission at best or by frank ridicule at worst, medical generation after generation is taught that the plumbing is all important and that all else is secondary. Attitudes such as these will have to change if alternative medicine is to play a valuable part in our society.

Second, the medical profession will have to come down from its pedestal and start accepting that it might not have all the answers. This will be the most difficult change to make, because public faith and adulation over the years have built doctors up to believe that they are much more able to cope with disease than in fact they are. A new humility and open-mindedness among the medical profession will mean listening to explanations offered by others, even if – horror of horrors – they are not doctors. The open-mindedness necessary to achieve this goal in any meaningful way looks a long way off unfortunately and may take two or three generations to come about.

Change is occurring slowly though, as was found in a 1984 study carried out for *The Times* newspaper in the UK. Some of the findings were rather surprising. For example:

1. 26 per cent of the doctors had tried a form of alternative medicine themselves for their own illness.

2. 57 per cent of those who were not already practising some kind of alternative therapy said that they would like to do so.

3. A much higher proportion of doctors actually practised some kind of alternative therapy than was previously thought and many more doctors referred patients to alternative practitioners than expected.

4. In spite of all this interest there was still 'wide-spread ignorance' of the therapies.

That all the GPs had heard of acupuncture and homoeopathy

comes as no surprise, but only one in six had heard of reflexology, and one in seven of the Alexander Technique. About 70 per cent of those questioned said that they recommended acupuncture, 48 per cent homoeopathy, 70 per cent hypnotherapy, and even 14 per cent healing. A growing number of GPs are opting for these therapies, because they find treatment with conventional therapies inappropriate for their patients or because their patients find them unsatisfactory.

All of this at first seems to be very good news for alternative medicine in general, and indeed it is. However, leaders in the field are concerned that just because someone is medically qualified doesn't mean that after a weekend course in, say, acupuncture they'll become an acupuncturist. The danger is that doctors, who, after all, have a training in a very particular sort of healing art, will see themselves as alternative practitioners after only minimal training. If they are properly trained (which, for most of the therapies, takes years) then this would, of course, be acceptable to everyone, but in Holland doctors wishing to train in an alternative therapy are excused only their basic medical science courses in any of the training schemes. This seems a sound idea if doctors are not to jump on the bandwagon of alternative medicine without the real understanding and change of thinking necessary to practise one of these healing arts successfully.

A fact that is frequently overlooked is that the medical profession is not the sole repository of knowledge when it comes to health matters. In the West it is simply the best organized, educated and vocal group, so doctors hold sway. Unfortunately, people are not going to be 'allowed' a wider spectrum of medical treatments unless and until the medical profession graciously agrees to it. Public opinion will help to bring about a change in this area in exactly the same way as it has done in the health food area – an area that started off with a few 'cranks' (who were simply way ahead of their time) and now embraces the food industry and is growing at an unforeseeable speed. I feel sure the same will occur with alternative therapies.

Since the first edition of this book alternative therapies have really taken off in the minds of the public all over the western world. This is none too surprising in the UK, with its liberal laws and fairly tame medical profession, but has taken everyone by storm in the US, where medical vested interests are powerful and vocal.

In December 1983 the Institute for Complementary Medicine in England conducted a survey into the natural therapies. A total of 1,800 alternative practitioners were circulated with a six-page questionnaire. Four hundred and eleven replied. The main findings were:

1. 163 practitioners named acupuncture as their main therapy, ninety-nine indicated chiropractic, thirty-three herbalism, twenty homoeopathy, fifteen naturopathy and seventy osteopathy.

2. Well over half the practitioners also used a second therapy and half the practitioners, a third. Virtually all had taken formal training in the therapies they practised, but a surprisingly large number had not joined any kind of Register.

3. For their main therapy 53 per cent of practitioners had trained full-time, 44 per cent had trained part-time and 44 per cent part-time by correspondence course.

4. There was a considerable variation between therapies, with, for example, 96 per cent of those offering chiropractic having trained full-time.

5. Despite the current demand for such therapies, only 33 per cent of the practitioners practised full-time.

6. The number of patients seen per week ranged from ten to 150, with chiropractors and osteopaths seeing on average about sixty patients a week. Extrapolating from these and other figures, the report suggests that there are about 4.6 million consultations with alternative medical therapists each year in the UK.

7. There are consistently more women than men consulting natural practitioners and the majority are in the twenty to thirty-nine and forty to fifty-nine age groups. Homoeopaths and herbalists tend to see more children than do the others.

8. Most therapists get their patients by word of mouth. Only

about 6 per cent of referrals came from general medical practitioners.

9. As to the number of consultations necessary, nearly half said that five to ten was the norm.

All of this shows just how the natural therapies are taking off in the UK, and there are no signs that this interest is abating – on the contrary, everything points to an ever-increasing public interest in the subject.

Third, practitioners of alternative medical therapies must be accepted and allowed to practise and do research. In the West they are relatively few in number and often poorly regarded, ignored or ridiculed, yet they find that they are in great public demand and have little time for research. This is a tremendous shame because what most of the alternative therapies need more than anything else are some properly conducted clinical trials that *prove* to everyone that they *do* work. Their practitioners *know* they work, because they see the results every day, but they find it well nigh impossible to prove that they do, except by anecdotal reports. As with so many things today the whole subject revolves around money. Orthodox medicine receives billions of dollars every year to set up theories, test them and report on the results. Almost no funds are available in the western world for research into fringe medicines so the research doesn't get done. It's a vicious circle. No money, no research. No research means you're a quack and quacks don't get given research monies.

What – no trials?

It is difficult to talk to orthodox doctors and scientists about alternative medical therapies for very long without their mentioning the importance of clinical trials to prove that any one therapy is valuable. In fact, I find that the shortage of trials in many of these fields is the greatest stumbling block to most medics. This is because doctors are brought up to believe that a treatment can only be considered valid if it has been proved to be so in trials.

There are many different sorts of clinical trial but basically they can be either 'controlled' or 'uncontrolled'. In the latter, the therapist simply logs all the results of a particular treatment and then analyses how successful or otherwise the treatment seems to have been. Controlled trials set much more rigid rules, classify the patients being treated, use placebos and may involve a situation in which neither the doctor nor the patient knows which treatment is being given. This last type of trial is held by many to be the best because, they claim, there can be no bias.

Certainly, such trials are effective when assessing drugs but are probably either impossible or extremely difficult to carry out with alternative medical therapies, because, by their very definition, most of the natural therapies treat each patient as a unique individual and not simply as another case of high blood pressure'! To most alternative therapists the idea of grouping patients with, for example, high blood pressure together and treating them all in exactly the same way is unthinkable – simply because the underlying causes for the disease may be different in each individual.

But if double-blind or similar sophisticated trial methods can't be done with these alternative therapies, why can't there simply be properly controlled trials, the medical world asks. This is a fair comment but one which in many ways poses the same question, because the very nature of many of the alternative medical therapies makes controlled trials difficult. If you're working with intuition, psychic forces and other unmeasurable parameters you can't control the therapy carefully enough to be able to repeat it exactly on another occasion. The difficulties of achieving this will become apparent to readers as they read each entry. Anyway there is a very strong case to be made for using the output from completely uncontrolled clinical trials as acceptable evidence. In other words, if a thing seems to work repeatedly – it works!

Having said this, trials have been done on various alternative and natural therapies and new trials are just about to start (1985) on spiritual healing in the treatment of painful conditions. The conditions and the patients are being chosen by doctors and 'easy' ailments are being excluded.

Dr Cyril Maxwell (medical adviser to an international pharmaceutical company) explained the problems with double-blind trials very well in a letter to the *British Medical Journal* in 1971. He took as his example the use of the drug imipramine in the management of nocturnal bed wetting in children. His research showed that early on in the history of this treatment the controlled trials showed imipramine not to be valuable. One trial in 1962 found the drug not to be useful; two further trials in 1963 were negative (although a further one was positive); but by 1964 controlled trials were showing that the drug was useful and not useful in equal numbers of publications. From then on papers appeared regularly proving that imipramine was in fact useful. Over the next five years fifteen papers appeared 'proving' its usefulness and one 'proving' its uselessness. Had the 'proof' before 1964 been adopted as final, a perfectly valuable treatment, as judged by previously uncontrolled clinical trials, would have been lost. Dr Maxwell's point is that just because a trial in medicine is controlled, this does not necessarily make it a good or valid one. All the trials with the bed wetters would have been considered well controlled but previously conducted uncontrolled trials still came up with the right answer . . . and sooner. Other controlled trials (nineteen in all) of the same drug but this time for the treatment of depression did no more than confirm the findings (fourteen years before in an uncontrolled trial) that it was effective in the treatment of depression.

So it seems important to me to value uncontrolled trials done by honest people with good intent, at least as a starting point for further research. Certainly, a new treatment should never be ignored or ridiculed simply because it hasn't undergone the most rigorous trials we can think of. Had this been the case in orthodox medicine, many very useful drugs would have been denied us – just as we *are* being denied many of the alternative therapies.

Orthodox medics are beginning to accept this point of view, albeit patchily and slowly. Recent research on feverfew has shown that it is just as powerful as modern anti-inflammatory, non-steroidal drugs, yet no one knows what the active ingredient is, so it can't be synthesized. A writer in the *Lancet* suggested that western doctors should use whole plants if they could be shown to work, rather than waiting for scientists to isolate the active ingredients and then make them into medicines.

Even when trials are adequately carried out (and they're difficult to do in many fringe medicines, because the varieties of treatments are often so much more numerous than those of orthodox medicine – see especially Herbal Medicine, page 162) orthodox medics are loath to take them seriously and quite understandably (though inexcusably) feel threatened if the results should prove the therapy valuable.

The medical profession appears to be desperately insecure – and with good reason. It cannot accept criticism or discussion, especially when it comes from outside the profession. Yet in countries as vast as China and Africa traditional medicine works side by side with the best of modern medicine and each has a respect for the other, because there are areas best suited to each and areas where the other should keep out.

Nowhere has this unwillingness of the medical profession to open itself up to criticism been more clearly exemplified than in the British Medical Association's inquiry into alternative medicines. There is understandably considerable concern among natural therapists about this inquiry, because the BMA (the UK doctors' trade union) has very obvious vested interests in keeping things as they are. No member of the inquiry has any apparent qualifications in any of the natural therapies and, because the BMA appears to be acting as judge and jury in the matter, many of the representatives of the leading natural therapies have refused to give evidence. Most people in the natural therapies fear that the BMA inquiry will be unable to recommend the majority of the therapies and will only endorse others when practised by doctors or by trained lay practitioners working under the supervision of doctors. Not surprisingly, the average natural therapist who spends much of his time 'picking up the pieces' that orthodox medicine has dropped doesn't want to become a handmaiden to a doctor like a physiotherapist or a chiropodist.

By the time this book is published the inquiry will have reported – at least everyone hopes so after such a long delay. Things have been so protracted that many in the natural health field wonder if there will ever be a publication.

Alternative medicine around the world

Traditional medicine exists in all cultures to some degree and terms such as 'indigenous medicine' or 'folk medicine' are used to describe such practices. Traditional medicine dates back hundreds or even thousands of years, depending on the country and culture concerned. Because two-thirds of the world's population (mainly in the developing countries) relies entirely on such traditional medical therapies, the World Health Organization has declared its intention actively to encourage traditional medicine worldwide in order that their goal of 'health for all by the year 2000' can be attained. It's interesting that even where western medical care is available, the majority of the people in the Third World chooses to remain loyal to its indigenous medical system, be it Ayurveda, Chinese, Siddha or Unani. The WHO has pledged itself to 'foster a realistic approach to traditional medicine; to explore the merits of traditional medicine in the lights of modern science in order to discourage harmful practices and encourage useful ones; and to promote the integration of proven valuable knowledge and skills in traditional and western medicine'. And, claims one WHO report, 'For far too long traditional systems of medicine and "modern" medicine have gone their separate ways in mutual antipathy. Yet are not their goals identical – to improve the health of mankind and thereby the quality of life? Only the blinkered mind would assume that each has nothing to learn from the other.'

It's all too easy to assume that the WHO need only concern itself with underdeveloped countries, but this is far from the case. Just as these poorer countries cannot afford western medicine, there are signs that we may not be able to much longer either. The very same pressures that apply in the Third World also apply, albeit to a lesser degree, to us in the West. To assume that because we are rich we can squander our wealth on unnecessarily expensive health care is rash in the extreme and we owe it to ourselves to look for ways of achieving the same end result more cheaply.

Almost every country has its own traditional medical system. For the Chinese it is acupuncture; for the French, magnetic healing; for the Germans, *Heilpraxis*; for the British, herbalism; with bone setting common to most. But along with folklore and superstition came quackery and this led the medical establishment to attempt to stifle and suppress folk medicine in the past. People naturally assumed that newer and more expensive medical care must be better and, guided by the medical profession, they were brainwashed into believing that anything that was not orthodox western medicine was either harmful or useless. This led to legislation which controls the practice of medicine by people who are not doctors in most countries.

The legal status of practitioners of alternative medical therapies varies enormously around the world. In the USA you have to be a medical doctor to be an osteopath, and after many lawsuits chiropractors, until recently outside the law, are now registered. Lay acupuncturists are outlawed in several states, yet people continue to go to them. Some provinces of Canada have naturopathic, chiropractic and osteopathic laws. In North America, unless laws specifically permit the practice of alternative medical therapies, they are illegal, yet alternative medicine is booming as nowhere else. The exact opposite applies in the UK, where, under Common Law, anyone can set themselves up as a therapist in anything providing they don't pretend to be a medical doctor. This has meant that over the years alternative medicine has flourished in the UK simply because it is so easy to practise there. 'Patients' of these practitioners have recourse to the law should anything go wrong and the system seems to work very well. Such a system is improved upon only by Western Germany, which has a licensing system for its alternative therapists (*Heilpraktikers*) of whom there are 3,700. These are healers or other fringe medical practitioners who are licensed by the state. They are screened to ensure that they are not a public danger and that they are socially responsible.

About twenty years ago India decided that greater priority should be given to traditional medicine and under the legislative scheme now in force there, practitioners of orthodox medicine and the traditional systems are registered under the same statute. It is specifically laid down that all medical training be based on the concept of the whole individual and not the part. Every student takes a basic course in anatomy, physiology, biology and pathology. Thereafter, they take the specialist course of their choice, whether modern western medicine, homoeopathic, ayurvedic or unani, and all qualified (registered) practitioners are on an equal footing. The Indian system contrasts with the two-tier West German system under which the *Heilpraktikers* (alternative practitioners) are licensed under a different statute from the one under which the doctors are registered.

The situation in Australia until recently followed UK lines. Legislation is currently under way though in the state of Victoria to regulate alternative medical practice and it looks as though everything except osteopathy and chiropractic will be declared illegal and that even these will have to be practised under strict medical control. As the rest of Australia usually follows the leadership of a key state such as Victoria, it looks as though fringe medicine will be in for a hard time in Australia before long.

South Africa could easily have gone the same way when legislation was drawn up in 1974. South Africa started out with a totally repressive attitude but was swayed by considerable evidence from around the world and brought in two Acts, one for homoeopathic, osteopathic, naturopathic and herbal medicine practitioners and the other for chiropractors. Under the first Act, practically anything reasonable was acceptable.

Much of continental Europe is governed by the old principle of Napoleonic Law that broadly excludes anything that hasn't actually been declared legal. In these countries only doctors and medical auxiliaries may practise medicine legally. France, for example, has no laws permitting fringe medical practice (except by doctors) but nevertheless tolerates the presence of 18,000 *guérisseurs* (healers), who are in constant demand by the public. The occasional complaint by a doctor or a patient will lead to a technical infringement of the law, but action is hardly ever taken. The Dutch, the Canton of Appenzel in Switzerland (the rest of Switzerland permits only chiropractic), the Swedes, Belgians and Norwegians are tolerant of fringe practitioners, who, as in France, are practising illegally. Because of this state of affairs, orthodox doctors on the continent of Europe are much more likely to be practising radiesthesia, for example, simply because there is a public demand which others are not allowed to satisfy.

Most of the emerging African nations encourage traditional and fringe medicines but, as mentioned above, the best example of both orthodox and traditional working side by side is to be found in China. In 1949, the existing health services were scant and couldn't serve a fraction of the country's vast needs. By integrating traditional and western medical systems and then by training primary health care workers, popularly known as 'barefoot doctors', the whole country quickly enjoyed remarkable health care. The whole population is involved in health care and people are taught to look after themselves – a mass movement which has eliminated their four great pests, rats, fleas, mosquitoes and bed bugs.

It is surprising to many people that the USA doesn't lead the world in alternative medical therapies, given as it is to experimenting with new ideas and to promoting advances effectively and quickly. The situation is very complex though, with laws differing from state to state with regard to any one therapy. Osteopathy, which involves a longer training than that for orthodox medicine, is widely accepted by law; every state has legislated in favour of chiropractic; and naturopathy is permitted in thirteen states. The American medical profession has, until recently, been hostile towards alternative therapies (or wholistic medicine, as it is called in the USA because it deals with the whole person), but is now softening in the presence of enormous public interest and considerable legal pressure from alternative practitioners. Scarcely a week goes by without a major television programme, magazine article or press report expressing disenchantment with orthodox medicine as practised in the USA and looking towards a more human approach. With the growth of interest in environmental matters and ecology, the American public is turning to its internal environment and is more aware than ever of the importance of healthy living.

As alternative therapies have been under a cloud for so long in the USA, there is now real excitement in the air and great hopes that legislation will be modified substantially in the not too distant future. There is good reason to suppose that this might occur as many of the top officials in the Department of Health, Education and Welfare are in favour of wholistic medicine, as was borne out at a major conference on the subject in Washington DC which was opened by one of them. Ex-President Carter himself has a sister who is a healer and he is reported to be open to wholistic medicine. The American Medical Association has taken no official position on the subject, but a spokesman, when asked for its standpoint, reportedly said that the AMA was 'in favour of wholistic medicine just as it is in favour of motherhood'. This rather cold stance is slowly being softened as increasing numbers of younger physicians are showing an interest in the natural therapies. Ten years from now the situation will be unrecognizably better.

A powerful lobby against the growth of alternative therapies would probably be the pharmaceutical industry. This rich and by and large highly responsible section of industry makes its money providing the public with what it thinks it needs – rather like General Motors supplies cars. The fact that some people kill themselves in cars doesn't stop GM making them nor should it, and likewise the occurrence of thalidomide tragedies and the high level of side-effects of drugs shouldn't, and won't, stop drug companies researching and manufacturing new and better products. It is very easy to see how the drug companies might feel if a new wave of interest were to arise in non-drug-orientated natural therapies. However, the innovative and ethical companies would find ways of replacing lost revenue from the market place and would soon be back where they were financially. The pharmaceutical industry has wrongly been labelled as the rogue of the piece of orthodox western medicine. This is unfair. People have a choice and our western society depends on them exerting their choice. *The trouble is that people are free to choose how they make themselves ill but not how they make themselves well.*

This is a book about what choices there are. None of the therapies mentioned will be available everywhere but the general trend throughout the western world is for them to spread. If your personal contacts don't lead you to the kind of therapy you want to try – you can seek help from a doctor or from other health sources. Some of the alternative therapies have official bodies and in the UK, for example, the Institute of Complementary Medicine in London keeps a directory of practitioners of the leading organizations so that the public and the medical profession can easily find out where their nearest therapist is. It's often a good idea when trying to select a practitioner to get in contact with one of these governing bodies. Magazines abound on the subject of health and healthy living and sometimes the adverts can lead you to the therapist you need. Hopefully the day is not far off when you will be able to go openly and without fear of any stigma attached to an alternative medical therapist of your choice. There are signs that this is, in fact, occurring and has been doing so with increasing speed since the first edition of this book. Research shows that many doctors are happy to refer patients to natural therapists practising in one of the five or six main areas and that they actively use them themselves when they are ill. Having said this, there *is* still a stigma to going to an alternative therapist and many people keep their visits a secret from their doctor in case the doctor is upset. I think this is a shame. First, because doctors should be made aware that the treatment they are using isn't working, and second, because if the individual gets better as a result of a natural therapist's efforts the medical doctors could erroneously imagine that *their* therapy was the cause. By shielding doctors from what they want and what they do, the average member of the public perpetuates the divide between the two systems of medicine. Almost any doctor has a list of horror stories of what has happened to patients at the hands of the dreaded 'quacks' but few have a list of the 'alternative' successes where they, the doctors, have failed.

Of course it is up to you to satisfy yourself that you're not dealing with a quack. There are charlatans in the fringe medicine world just as there are inside medicine. There are also all shades of opinion even within any given area of alternative medicine. Much as with orthodox medicine, it depends on whom you see to a great extent. Be guided by personal recommendation whenever possible and if you can find doctors who specialize in or even have a sideline in the fringe medicine you want, I think it's worth going to them. The chances are that their deeper knowledge of a wider range of medical facts will make them better at assessing the problem in the first place. The actual treatment part is not *necessarily* best carried out by a medically qualified person. Doctors certainly don't have a monopoly of healing powers. In fact, the gift of healing is very widespread – much more so than is generally realized – and many priests and even ordinary members of the public have powers of healing. Good doctors should not only be able to manipulate modern medical knowledge to the patient's advantage but should also be good healers. Non-medical healers can be equally successful if given a chance. Indeed, millions of people the world over fare very well in the hands of such non-medical healers.

I have tried to be as honest and straightforward as possible about each subject included in this book. All of the methods have something to offer and many of them can offer a great deal if given a chance. Where they seem to be useless as assessed by things we *can* understand, it is indicated. However, conclusions of this sort may not always prove to be correct. For example, I've tried to explain how acupuncture and homoeopathy work in terms of our modern knowledge of physiology and nuclear chemistry respectively. It may be that the way they really work is quite different, but I can only explain things within the bounds of what is known and acceptable in today's world. The reader should bear in mind that doctors don't really know how lots of orthodox medical treatments work, yet we happily use them year after year on millions of people. For example, it wasn't known how aspirin worked until about fifteen years ago, yet that didn't stop it being the most widely used medicine in the world for over seventy years.

People are going to have to change their attitudes to unorthodox forms of medicine. Every year that goes by opens new doors to our understanding of the human mind and body and as this happens we understand a little more of how one of the 'way-out', 'cranky' medical treatments works. In the meantime it would be disastrous to throw the baby out with the bath water and with typical western arrogance dismiss something because it's 'unproven' or 'difficult to explain'.

The turning point will only come when alternative medical therapies are considered as first line treatments in their own right and not as they are today in the West – the final resting place of the 'garbage' untreatable by the medical profession. As western medicine is accepted by the developing world, more of the world's population gets the best of both traditional and western medical systems. Why shouldn't we in the West have the same privilege?

Further Reading

Since this book was last printed certain parts of the reading list have been expanded to favour the most widely available alternative therapies. Two new sections, Approaches to Cancer and Relaxation and Stress Management, have been added.

Acupuncture

AUSTIN, M., *Acupuncture Therapy*, Thorsons, Wellingborough, Northants, 1974

BLATE, M., *The Natural Healer's Acupressure Handbook*, Routledge & Kegan Paul, London, 1976

CHAITOW, L., *The Acupuncture Treatment of Pain*, Thorsons, Wellingborough, Northants, 1976

CONNELLY, D. M., *Traditional Acupuncture: The Law of the Five Elements*, Center for Traditional Acupuncture, Columbia, Maryland, 1979

Essentials of Chinese Acupuncture, Foreign Languages Press, Beijing, 1980

KAPTCHUK, T. J., *Chinese Medicine: The Web That Has No Weaver*, Hutchinson, London, 1983

KENYON, J. N., *Modern Techniques in Acupuncture Vols I and II*, Thorsons, Wellingborough, Northants, 1983

LAWSON-WOOD, D. and LAWSON-WOOD, J., *First Aid at Your Fingertips*, Daniel, Saffron Walden, Essex, 1963

LEE, J. F. and CHEUNG, C. S., *Current Acupuncture Therapy*, Medical Book Publications, Hong Kong, 1978

LEWITH, G. T. and LEWITH, N. R., *Modern Chinese Acupuncture*, Thorsons, Wellingborough, Northants, 1980

MACDONALD, A., *Acupuncture from Ancient Art to Modern Medicine*, Unwin Paperbacks, London, 1982

MANAKA, Y. and URQUART, A., *The Layman's Guide to Acupuncture*, Weatherhill, New York, 1972

MANN, F., *Acupuncture: The Ancient Chinese Art of Healing*, Random House, New York, 1973

NOGIER, P. F. M., *From Auriculotherapy to Auriculomedicine*, Maisonneuve, Sainte-Ruffine, 1983

O'CONNOR, J. and BENSKY, D., *Acupuncture: A Comprehensive Text*, Eastland Press, Seattle, Washington, 1981

An Outline of Chinese Acupuncture, Academy of Traditional Chinese Medicine, Foreign Languages Press, Beijing, 1975

PAINE, D. L. S., *Acupuncture, Traditional Diagnosis and Treatment*, East Asia Co, London, 1984

PORKERT, M., *The Theoretical Foundations of Chinese Medicine*, MIT Press, Cambridge, Mass, 1974

VEITH, I., *The Yellow Emperor's Classic of Internal Medicine*, University of California Press, Berkeley, 1949

Alexander Technique

ALEXANDER, F. M., *The Alexander Technique: The Essential Writings of F. Mathias Alexander*, Thames and Hudson, London, 1974

ALEXANDER, F. M., *Constructive Conscious Control*, Centerline Press, Downey, California, 1985

ALEXANDER, F. M., *The Use of Self*, Centerline Press, Downey, California, 1984

BARKER, S., *The Alexander Technique: The Revolutionary Way to Use Your Body for Total Energy*, Bantam Books, New York, 1978

BARLOW, W., *The Alexander Principle: How to Use Your Body*, Arrow Books, London, 1975

BARLOW, W., *More Talk of Alexander*, Gollancz, London, 1978

BYLES, M. B., *Stand Straight without Strain*, Fowler, Romford, Essex, 1978

FENTON, J. V., *Practical Movement Control*, Plays Inc, New York, 1973

GELB, M., *Body Learning: An Introduction to the Alexander Technique*, Aurum Press, London, 1983

JONES, F. P., *Body Awareness in Action: A Study of the Alexander Technique*, Schocken Books, New York, 1979

Anthropsophical Medicine

STEINER, R., *Spiritual Science and Medicine*, Steiner Publishing Co., London, 1948

DAVY, J. (ed), *Work Arising from the Life of Rudolph Steiner*, Rudolph Steiner Press, London, 1975

Aromatherapy

ARNOULD-TAYLOR, W. E., *Aromatherapy for the Whole Person*, Arnould-Taylor Education Ltd and Stanley Thornes Ltd, Cheltenham, Glos, 1981

LAUTIÉ, R. and PASSEBECQ, A., *Aromatherapy: The Use of Plant Essences in Healing*, Thorsons, Wellingborough, Northants, 1979

MAURY, M., *The Secret of Life and Youth*, MacDonald, London, 1964 (currently out of print but soon to be republished as *The Madame Maury Guide to Aromatherapy*, Daniel, Saffron Walden, Essex)

PRICE, S., *Practical Aromatherapy: The Use of Essential Oils for Restoring Vitality*, Thorsons, Wellingborough, Northants, 1983

RYMAN, D., *The Aromatherapy Handbook*, Century Publishing, London, 1984

TISSERAND, M., *Aromatherapy for Women*, Thorsons, Wellingborough, Northants, 1985

TISSERAND, R. B., *The Art of Aromatherapy*, Daniel, Saffron Walden, Essex, 1977

TISSERAND, R. B., *Essential Oils: Safety Date Manual*, Association of Aromatherapists, Brighton, East Sussex, 1985

VALNET, J., *Practice of Aromatherapy*, Daniel, Saffron Walden, Essex, 1980

Ayurveda

THAKKUR, C., *Introduction to Ayurveda*, ASI Publishers Inc., New York, 1974

Bach Remedies

WEEKS, N. and BULLEN, V., *The Bach Flower Remedies*, Daniel, Saffron Walden, Essex, 1964

Biochemics

CHAPMAN, E., *How to Use the Twelve Tissue Salts*, Pyramid, New York, 1977

Biofeedback and Autogenic Training

BASMAJIAN, J. V., *Biofeedback: Principles and Practice for Clinicians*, Williams and Wilkins, Baltimore, 1983

BLUNDELL G., *EEG Measurement: A Study in Depth of Brain Wave-patterns and their Significance*, Audio Ltd, London

BROWN, B., *New Mind, New Body*, Bantam Books, New York, 1975

COXHEAD, N. and CADE, M., *The Awakened Mind: Biofeedback and the Development of Higher States of Awareness*, Wildwood House, London, 1980

DANSKIN, D. and CROW, M., *Biofeedback: An Introduction and Guide*, Mayfield Publishing Co, California, 1981

FULLER, G. D., *Biofeedback Methods and Procedure in Clinical Practice*, Biofeedback Institute of San Francisco, 1977

GRATCHEL, R. J., *Clinical Application of Biofeedback: Appraisal and Status*, Pergamon Press, Oxford, 1979

GREEN, E. and GREEN A., *Beyond Biofeedback, Delacorte Press, New York, 1977*

HUME, W. I. (ed), *Biofeedback: Annual Research Review, Vol 3*, Human Sciences Press, New York, 1981

KAMIYA, J. (ed), *Biofeedback and Self Control (Annuals)*, Aldine Atherton Publishing Co, Chicago, 1970–77

KARLINS, M. and ANDREWS, L. M., *Biofeedback: Turning on the Power of Your Mind*, Abacus, London, 1975

KARLINS, M. and ANDREWS, L. M., *Man Controlled*, Free Press, New York, 1972

LUTHE, W. and SHULTZ, J. H., *Autogenic Therapy, Vols 1–6*, Grune and Stratton, New York, 1969–73

OLTON, D. S. and NOONBERG, A. R., *Biofeedback: Clinical Applications in Behavioural Medicine*, Prentice Hall, London, 1980

POTELIAKHOFF, A. and CARRUTHERS, M., *Real Health*, Davis Poynter, London, 1981

ROHR, W. I., *Symptom Reduction through Clinical Biofeedback*, Human Sciences Press, New York, 1983

ROSA C., *You and Autogenic Training*, Dutton, New York, 1976

Chiropractic

CHAITOW, L., *Neuro-muscular Technique: A Practitioner's Guide to Soft Tissue Manipulation*, Thorsons, Wellingborough, Northants, 1980

CYRIAX, J., *Treatment by Manipulation, Massage and Injection*, Williams and Wilkins, Baltimore, 1971

54   *Alternative Medicine*

DINTENFUSS, J., *Chiropractic: A Modern Way to Health*, Pyramid Books, New York, 1973

JANSE, J., HOUSER, R. H. and WELLS, B. F. *Chiropractic Principles and Technique*, National College of Chiropractic, Chicago, 1947

KELNER, M., HALL, O. and COULTER, I., *Chiropractors: Do They Help?*, Fitzhenry and Whiteside, Toronto, 1980

LEACH, R. A., *The Chiropractic Theories: A Synopsis of Scientific Research*, Mid-South Scientific Publishers, Mississippi, 1980

MAITLAND, G. D., *Peripheral Manipulation*, Butterworth, London, 1970

MAITLAND, G. D., *Vertebral Manipulation*, Butterworth, London, 1964

PALMER, D. D. and PALMER, B. J., *The Science of Chiropractic: Its Principles and Adjustments*, Palmer School of Chiropractic, Davenport, Iowa, 1906

SCOFIELD, A. G., *Chiropractice: The Science of Specific Spinal Adjustment*, Thorsons, Wellingborough, Northants, 1968

Colour Therapy

HUNT, R., *Seven Keys to Colour Healing, Daniel, Saffron Walden, Essex, 1971*

BIRRON,, F., *Colour Psychology and Colour Therapy*, University Books, New Jersey, 1961

OTT, J. N., *Health and Light*, Pocket Books, Simon & Schuster, New York, 1976

Cymatics

JENNY, H., *Cymatics*, Basilius Prese, Basle, Vol I, 1967, Vol II, 1974

Do-In

DE LANGRE, J., *Do-In 2: The Ancient Art of Rejuvenation Through Self Massage*, Happiness Press, 160 Wycliff Way, Magalia, California, 1978

Healing

BAILEY, A. A., *Esoteric Healing: A Treatise on the Seven Rays*, Lucis Press, London, 1953

BLOOMFIELD, R., *The Mystique of Healing*, Skilton and Shaw, Edinburgh, 1984

CODDINGTON, M., *In Search of Healing Energy*, Thorsons, Wellingborough, Northants, 1981

COOKE, I., *Healing by the Spirit*, White Eagle Publishing Trust, Liss, Hants, 1976

EDWARDES, P. and MCCONNELL, J., *Healing for You*, Thorsons, Wellingborough, Northants, 1985

EDWARDS, H., *Guide to the Understanding and Practice of Spiritual Healing*, Healer Publishing Co Ltd, Burrows Lea, Guildford, Surrey, 1974

EDWARDS, H., *Healing Intelligence*, Healer Publishing Co Ltd, Burrows Lea, Guildford, Surrey, 1965

HARVEY, D., *The Power to Heal: An Investigation of Healing and the Healing Experience*, Aquarian Press, Wellingborough, Northants, 1983

LESHAN, L., *Clairvoyant Reality: Towards a General Theory of the Paranormal*, Turnstone Press, Wellingborough, Northants, 1974

LOOMIS, E. G. and PAULSON, J. S., *Healing for Everyone: Medicine of the Whole Person*, DeVorss and Co, Marine del Rey, California, 1975

MACMANAWAY, B. and TURCAN, J., *Healing: The Energy That Can Restore Health*, Thorsons, Wellingborough, Northants, 1983

MACNUTT, F., *Healing*, Corgi Books, London, 1977

MCALL, K., *Healing the Family Tree*, Sheldon Press, London, 1982

MEEK, G. W. (ed), *Healers and the Healing Process*, Theosophical Publishing House, Wheaton, Illinois, 1978

RAMACHARAHA, Yogi, *The Science of Psychic Healing*, Fowler and Co, Chadwell Heath, Essex, 1903

ST AUBYN, L. (ed), *Healing*, Heinemann, London, 1983

TESTER, M. H., *Healing Touch*, Psychic Press, London, 1970

THOMSON, W. A. R., *Faiths That Heal*, A. and C. Black, London, 1980

TRUNGPA, C., *Cutting Through Spiritual Materialism*, Shambala Publications Inc, Berkeley, California, 1973

Herbal Medicine

CLARKE, L., *Handbook of Natural Remedies for Common Ailments*, Thorsons, Wellingborough, Northants, 1976

CONWAY, D., *The Magic of Herbs*, Granada, London, 1973

CULPEPER, N. (ed POTTERTON, D.), *Culpeper's Colour Herbal*, W. Foulsham, Slough, Berks, 1983

DINCIN-BUCHMAN, D., *Herbal Medicine: The Natural Way to Get Well and Stay Well*, The Herb Society/Hutchinson, London, 1983

FLUCK, H., *Medicinal Plants and Their Uses*, W. Foulsham, Slough, Berks, 1976

GRIEVE, M., *A Modern Herbal*, Jonathan Cape, London, 1974

GRIGGS, B., *The Green Pharmacy: A History of Herbal Medicine*, Jill Norman and Hobhouse, London, 1981

HARPER-SHOVE, F., *Medicinal Herbs: Prescriber and Clinical Repertory*, Daniel, Saffron Walden, Essex, 1938

HOFFMAN, D., *The Holistic Herbal*, Findhorn Press, Findhorn, Moray, 1983

Hygieia: A Woman's Herbal, Wildwood House, Hounslow, Middlesex, 1979

KADANS, J. M., *Encyclopaedia of Medicinal Herbs*, Thorsons, Wellingborough, Northants, 1979

LEUNG, A., *Chinese Herbal Remedies*, Wildwood House, Hounslow, Middlesex, 1985

LEVY, J. de B., *Common Herbs for Natural Health?*, Schocken, New York, 1974

LUST, J., *The Herb Book*, Bantam Books, London, 1975

MESSEGUE, M., *Health Secrets of Plants and Herbs*, Collins, London, 1979

MITTON, F., and MITTON, V., *Mitton's Practical Modern Herbal*, W. Foulsham, Slough, Berks, 1976

SCHAUNBERG, P. and PARIS FERDINAND, P., *Guide to Medicinal Plants*, Lutterworth Press, Guildford, Surrey, 1977

THOMSON, W. A. R., *Healing Plants*, Macmillan, London, 1980

TIERRA, M., *The Way with Herbs*, Orenda/Unity Press, Santa Cruz, California, 1980

WREN, R. C., *Potter's New Cyclopaedia of Botanical Drugs and Preparations*, Daniel, Saffron Walden, Essex, 1907

Homoeopathy

BLACKIE, M. G., *The Patient, Not the Cure: The Challenge of Homoeopathy*, Unwin, London, 1981

BOERICKE and RUNYON, *The Principles of Homoeopathy*, 1896 (reprinted 1971 by Health Research, PO Box 70, Mobelumne Hill, California 95245)

CLOVER, A., *Homoeopathy: A Patient's Guide*, Thorsons, Wellingborough, Northants, 1984

DAY, C., *The Homoeopathic Treatment of Small Animals*, Wigmore Publications, London, 1984

GORDON ROSS, A. C., *Homoeopathy: An Introductory Guide*, Thorsons, Wellingborough, Northants, 1976

HAHNEMANN, S. (eds KUNKI, J., NAUDE, A. and PENDLETON, P.), *Organon of Medicine* (sixth edition, new translation), Gollancz, London, 1983

MACLEOD, G., *The Treatment of Horses by Homoeopathy*, Daniel, Saffron Walden, Essex, 1977

PANOS, M. B. and HEIMLICH, J., *Homoeopathic Medicine at Home*, Corgi Books, London, 1982

ROBERT, H. A., *The Principles and Art of Cure by Homoeopathy*, Daniel, Saffron Walden, Essex, 1936

SCOTT, K. and MCCOURT, L. A., *Homoeopathy*, Thorsons, Wellingborough, Northants, 1983

SHEPHERD, D., *Homoeopathy for the First Aider*, Daniel, Saffron Walden, Essex, 1972

SHEPHERD, D., *The Magic of the Minimum Dose*, Daniel, Saffron Walden, Essex, 1964

SPEIGHT, P., *A Comparison of the Chronic Miasms*, Daniel, Saffron Walden, Essex, 1961

STEPHENSON, J. H., *Helping Yourself with Homoeopathic Remedies*, Thorsons, Wellingborough, Northants, 1977

TYLER, M., *Homoeopathic Drug Pictures*, Daniel, Saffron Walden, Essex, 1942

VITHOULKAS, G., *Homoeopathy: Medicine of the New Man*, Arco Press, New York, 1980

WEINER, M. and GOSS, K., *The Complete Book of Homoeopathy*, Bantam Books, London, 1982

WHEELER, C. E. and KENYON, J. D., *Introduction to the Principles and Practice of Homoeopathy*, Daniel, Saffron Walden, Essex, 1980

Hydrotherapy *see* Naturopathy

Hypnosis

BLYTHE, P., *Self Hypnotism*, Barker, 1976

Macrobiotics

OHSAWA, G., *Practical Guide to Far Eastern Macrobiotic Medicine*. Published by George Ohsawa, Macrobiotic Foundation, 1544 Oak Street, Oroville, California 95965, 1973

Megavitamin Therapy

PFEIFFER, C. C., *Mental and Elemental Nutrients: A Physician's Guide to Nutrition and Health Care*, Keats, New Canaan, Connecticut, 1975

HAWKINS, D., and PAULING, L., *Orthomolecular Psychiatry*, Freeman, Reading and San Francisco, 1973

ADAMS, R. and MURRAY, F., *Megavitamin Therapy*, Larchmont Books, New York, 1974

Naturopathy and Hydrotherapy

AIROLA, P., *How to Get Well*, Health Plus Publishers, Phoenix, Arizona, 1974

BALANTINE, R., *Diet and Nutrition: A Holistic Approach,* The Himalayan International Institute, Honesdale, Pennsylvania, 1982

BIRCHER, R., *Eating Your Way to Health*, Faber, London, 1961

BLAND, J., *Medical Applications of Clinical Nutrition*, Keats Publishing Inc, New Canaan, Connecticut, 1983

DAVIES, A., *Let's Get Well*, George Unwin, London, 1984

Diets to Help, Thorsons, Wellingborough, Northants (a series of books giving diets which are beneficial to health problems such as acne, arthritis, catarrh, constipation, hay fever, heart disorders, liver complaints, psoriasis)

HOFFER, A., and WALKER, M., *Orthomolecular Nutrition*, Keats Publishers Inc, New Canaan, Connecticut, 1978

HOLFORD, P., *The Whole Food Guide to Elemental Health*, Thorsons, Wellingborough, Northants, 1983

JENSEN, B., *Nature Has a Remedy*, Unity Press, Santa Cruz, California, 1978

LEDERMAN, E. K., *The Common Sense Guidebook to a Healthier New Life*, Pan Books, London, 1976

LINDLAHR, H., *Natural Therapeutics* (3 vols), Daniel, Saffron Walden, Essex – ed PROBY, J., Vol 1. Philosophy, 1975; Vol 2. Practice, 1981; Vol 3. Natural Dietetics, 1983

MELLOR, C., *Constance Mellor's Natural Remedies for Common Ailments*, Granada, London, 1975

MERVYN, L., *Dictionary of Vitamins: The Complete Guide to Vitamins and Vitamin Therapy*, Thorsons, Wellingborough, Northants, 1984

NEWMAN-TURNER, R., *Naturopathic Medicine: Treating the Whole Person*, Thorsons, Wellingborough, Northants, 1984

PFEIFFER, C. C., *Mental and Elemental Nutrients: A Physician's Guide to Nutrition and Health Care*, Keats Publishing Inc, New Canaan, Connecticut, 1975

POWELL, E. F. W., *The Natural Home Physician*, Daniel, Saffron Walden, Essex, 1962

PRICE, W., *Nutrition and Physical Degeneration*, Price–Pottenger Foundation, California, 1945

WARMBRAND, M., *Encylopaedia of Health and Nutrition*, Pyramid Publishing, New York, 1974

WILLIAMS, R., *Nutrition against Disease*, Bantam Books, New York, 1973

WRIGHT, B., *Natural Healing with Herbal Combinations*, Green Press, Burwash, East Sussex, 1984

Negative Ion Therapy

SOYKA, S. and EDMONDS, A., *The Ion Effect*, Bantam, Dutton & Co., New York, 1978

Orgone Therapy

BOADELLA, B., *Wilhelm Reich: The Evolution of His Work*, Dell, New York, 1976

REICH, W., *The Orgone Accumulator: Its Medical and Scientific Use* (originally published by The Orgone Institute Press, Maine, 1951; reprinted by CORPS, Box 1956, c/o Rising Free, 182 Upper Street, London, N1)

Osteopathy

ASHMORE, E. F., *Osteopathic Mechanics*, Tamor Pierston Publications, Isleworth, Middlesex, 1981

BROOKES, D., *Lectures on Cranial Osteopathy*, Thorsons, Wellingborough, Northants, 1981

CHAITOW, L., *Neuro-muscular Technique: A Practitioner's Guide to Soft Tissue Manipulation*, Thorsons, Wellingborough, Northants, 1980

CHAITOW, L., *Osteopathy: A Complete Health Care System*, Thorsons, Wellingborough, Northants, 1982

CYRIAX, J., *Treatment by Manipulation, Massage and Injection*, Williams and Wilkins, Baltimore, 1971

LETTVEN M., *The Back Book: Healing the Hurt in Your Lower Back*, Souvenir Press, London, 1976

MAITLAND, G. D., *Peripheral Manipulation*, Butterworth, London, 1970

MAITLAND, G. D., *Vertebral Manipulation*, Butterworth, London, 1964

STODDARD, A., *The Back: Relief from Pain*, Martin Dunitz, London, 1979

STODDARD, A., *Manual of Osteopathic Practice*, Hutchinson, London, 1969

STODDARD, A., *Manual of Osteopathic Techniques*, Hutchinson, London, 1959

WHITE, A. A., *Your Aching Back*, Bantam Books, New York, 1983

Pattern Therapy *see* **Radiesthesia**

Psionic Medicine
REYNER, J. H., LAURENCE, G., and UPTON, C., *Psionic Medicine: The Study and Treatment of the Causative Factors in Illness*, Routledge & Kegan Paul, London, 1974

Pyramid Therapy
FLANAGAN, G. P., *Pyramid Power*, De Vorss & Co., Los Angeles, 1973
KERRELL, B. and GOGGIN, K., *The Guide to Pyramid Energy*, Pyramid Power, V. Inc., California, 1975

Radiesthesia and Pattern Therapy
WESTLAKE, A. T., *The Pattern Health*, Shambhala, Berkeley and London, 1973
BELL, A. H., *Practical Dowsing*, Bell & Sons, London, 1965

Radionics
TANSLEY, D. V., *Radiation and the Subtle Anatomy of Man*, Health Science Press, Devon, 1972
RUSSELL, E. W., *Report on Radionics*, Spearman, Sudbury, Suffolk, 1973

Reflexology
INGHAM, E. D., *Stories the Feet Can Tell: Stepping to Better Health*, Ingham Publishing, PO Box 8412, Rochester, New York, NY 14618, 1959
INGHAM, E. D., *Stories the Feet Have Told*, Ingham Publishing, PO Box 8412, Rochester, New York, NY 14618, 1959

Rolfing
ROLF, I., *Rolfing: Structural Integration*, Landman, San Francisco, 1977
JOHNSON, D., *Protean Body: A Rolfer's View of Human Flexibility*, Harper & Row, New York, 1977

Shiatsu
NAMIKOSHI, I., *Shiatsu Therapy and Practice*, Japan Publications Inc., Tokyo, 1974

Yoga
RAMACHARAKA, *Hatha Yoga – or the Yogi Philosophy of Physical Well Being*, Fowler, Romford, Essex, 1917
FUNDERBURK, J., *Science Studies Yoga*, Himalayan International Institute of Yoga Science and Philosophy of the USA, 1977

General Background Interest

BURR, H. S. *Blueprint for Immortality*, Spearman, Sudbury, Suffolk, 1972

COXHEAD, N., *Mindpower: The Emerging Pattern of Current Research*, Heinemann, London, 1976

DE CHARDIN, P. T., *The Phenomenon of Man*, Fontana, Collins, London, 1959

FORBES, A., *Try Being Healthy*, Langdon Books, Plymouth, 1976

KARAGULLA, S., *Breakthrough to Creativity*, De Vorss & Co., Los Angeles, 1977

KERVRAN, C. L., *Biological Transmutations*, Crosby Lockwood, London, 1971

MACKARNESS, R., *Not All in the Mind*, Pan Books, London, 1976

PLAYFAIR, G. L. and HILL, S., *The Cycles of Heaven*, Souvenir, London, 1978

STELTER, A., *Psi-healing*, Bantam, New York, 1976

TOMPKINS, P. and BIRD, C., *The Secret Life of Plants*, Harper & Row, London, 1973

WATSON, L., *Supernature*, Hodder, London, 1973; Doubleday, New York, 1973

Approaches to Cancer

AIROLA, P. O., *Cancer: Causes, Prevention and Treatment – The Total Approach*, Health Plus Publications, Phoenix, Arizona, 1972

BISHOP, B., *A Time to Heal*, Severn House Publishers, London, 1985

CAMERON, E. and PAULING, L., *Cancer and Vitamin C*, Warner Books, New York, 1981

CHAITOW, L., *An End to Cancer?*, Thorsons, Wellingborough, Northants, 1983

FERE, M. T., *Does Diet Cure Cancer?*, Thorsons, Wellingborough, Northants, 1963

FORBES, A., *The Bristol Diet: A Get Well and Stay Well Eating Plan*, Century Publishing, London, 1984

GERSON, M., *A Cancer Therapy: Results of Fifty Cases*, Totality Books, Del Mar, California, 1958

HALSTEAD, B. W., *Metabolic Cancer Therapy*, Golden Quill Publishers, Cotton, California, 1978

HOLMES, D., *New Hope and Improved Treatments for Cancer Patients*, distributed by John Wiley & Sons, Chichester, West Sussex, 1982

HORTA, R. A., *Physician's Handbook of Vitamin B-17 Therapy*, C & R Internacional, Tijuana, 1978

KIDMAN, B., *A Gentle Way with Cancer*, Century Books, London, 1985

KUSHI, M., *The Cancer Prevention Diet*, Thorsons, Wellingborough, Northants, 1984

LESHAN, L., *You Can Fight for Your Life: Emotional Factors in the Treatment of Cancer*, Thorsons, Wellingborough, Northants, 1977

NEWBOLD, H. L., *Vitamin C against Cancer*, Stein and Day Publishers, New York, 1979

PEARCE, I., *The Gate of Healing*, Neville Spearman, Jersey, Channel Islands, 1983

SIMONTON, O. C., MATTHEWS-SIMONTON, S. and CREIGHTON, J. L., *Getting Well Again*, Bantam Books, New York, 1980

Relaxation and Stress Management

BENSON, H. and KLIPPER, M. Z., *The Relaxation Response*, William Collins, London, 1976

CHAITOW, L., *Your Complete Stress-Proofing Programme: How to Protect Yourself Against the Ill Effects of Stress*, Thorsons, Wellingborough, Northants, 1983

CHARLESWORTH, E. A. and NATHAN, G. N., *Stress Management: A Comprehensive Guide to Wellness*, Stress Management Associates, Houston, Texas, 1981

COLEMAN, V., *Stress and Your Stomach*, Sheldon Press, London, 1983

CURTIS, J. and DETERT, R., *How to Relax: A Holistic Approach to Stress Management*, Mayfield Publishing Co, California, 1981

FINK, D., *Release from Nervous Tension*, Allen & Unwin, Hemel Hempstead, Herts, 1967

HEWITT, J., *Nature's Way with Tension*, Thorsons, Wellingborough, Northants, 1968

LAKE, T., *How to Cope with Your Nerves*, Sheldon Press, London, 1982

Living with Stress, Consumers' Association, London, 1982

MADDERS, J., *Stress and Relaxation: Self-Help Ways to Cope with Stress and Relieve Nervous Tension, Ulcers, Insomnia, Migraine and High Blood Pressure*, Martin Dunitz, London, 1979

PELLETIER, K., *Mind as Healer, Mind as Slayer: A Holistic Approach to Preventing Stress Disorders*, Allen & Unwin, London, 1978

QUICK, C., *Diets to Help Hypertension*, Thorsons, Wellingborough, Northants, 1978

SELYE, H., *The Stress of Life*, McGraw Hill, New York, 1978

SHARPE, R. and LEWIS, D., *Thrive on Stress: How to Make It Work to Your Advantage*, Souvenir Press, London, 1977
TYRER, P., *How to Cope with Stress*, Sheldon Press, London, 1982
TYRER, P., *How to Sleep Better*, Sheldon Press, London, 1982
WEEKES, C., *Self-Help with Your Nerves*, Angus & Robertson, London, 1962

Caution

This is not a self-help book. The therapies outlined are only safe in the hands of experienced practitioners and none should be tried by the reader himself.

Wherever I have suggested that a particular therapy has been shown to be useful in a specific medical condition or group of conditions, I cannot promise the reader that it will produce the desired results in him. With western medicine such a promise would be similarly unwise.

If you have a medical problem, first consult your doctor and if he and his colleagues cannot help, then go to an alternative medical practitioner but preferably to one who also has an orthodox medical training.

Acupuncture

Definition

Acupuncture is a therapy based on the principle that there is a nervous connection between the organs of the body and the body surface. When an organ is diseased, acupuncture points, as they are called, appear in or just beneath the skin and are tender. The sufferer sometimes feels the tender spot or spots himself or may only realize they are there when a skilled practitioner presses over the point. Acupuncturists hold that these tender points disappear on treatment no matter how the patient is treated (either conventionally, homoeopathically or by acupuncture, for instance). Acupuncture itself involves the stimulation of these so-called acupuncture points, usually with fine needles, in such a way as to modify the activity of the point and so influence other parts of the body.

Background

Acupuncture is an ancient Chinese art dating back to the stone age. It is said that as long ago as 3000 BC the Chinese noticed that soldiers wounded with arrows sometimes got relief from diseases which had been troubling them for years. Whether this is true or not, it led the Chinese to evolve a system of medicine which cured diseases by penetrating the skin at specific points.

The word acupuncture literally means to puncture (punctura) with a needle (acus) but needles are not essential instruments and stone chips were used in antiquity. Rural Africans are said to have cures that involve scratching certain specific areas of the body; some Eskimos use sharp stones; and an isolated cannibalistic Brazilian tribe blows tiny arrows into the acupuncture points with a blowpipe.

Iron needles were used in the Iron Age but even before that sticks and thorns were the sole instruments of this new type of medicine. By 2900 BC it was thought that different metals used in the needles seemed to have different effects. It is now known that this isn't the case. We now know that the nature of the needle is unimportant compared with the way in which it is used. The needles used in acupuncture today are made of stainless steel so that they can be readily sterilized.

Although acupuncture is a system of medicine as old as Man himself, it was the Chinese who systematized it and wrote the first book on the subject in about 200 BC. This *Hungdi Neiging Suwen* (the Yellow Emperor's Classic in Internal Disease) is still widely referred to and contains many medical truths that are as applicable today as when they were written.

Acupuncture has since spread throughout the world but is still most widely practised in China and the Far East where medical students study either western medicine or traditional Chinese medicine at the same university.

In some Chinese hospitals, doctors from both disciplines will practise together, with a surgeon trained in western medicine performing an operation on a patient under acupuncture analgesia and with traditional doctors preventing post-operative pneumonia and urine retention. Very rarely an individual doctor practises both medical forms. It's ironic that the Chinese are beginning to take acupuncture and traditional Chinese medicine for granted (possibly to the point of underrating it) at the very time when we in the West are waking up to its potential. They wrongly assume that technological medicine will answer their problems in the way that other western technology has.

Today there are hundreds of acupuncturists in the West although in most countries they are still considered to be very much on the fringe of medicine.

What is it?

Acupuncture works on the principle that in all diseases, be they mental or physical, there are tender areas at certain points on the body which disappear when the disease is cured. These are called acupuncture points. Sometimes the patient will complain spontaneously that they are tender and sometimes that they are tender only on pressure. At other times these points may only be found with difficulty by a skilled practitioner of acupuncture. An acupuncture point may be a nodule (rather like the nodules found in fibrositis); a piece of tense muscle; or simply a tender area in the skin that may also be swollen and even discoloured.

The Chinese describe about 1,000 acupuncture points, some of which are recognized by orthodox medicine but aren't called by the same names. It's well known to doctors that disease in an organ can produce pain or tenderness and sometimes even skin changes in an area a long way from the affected organ. For instance, a painful condition near the diaphragm can produce pain in the shoulder tip. This is because the nerve supply to both areas has some elements in common and the brain is 'fooled' into thinking that pain from one is in fact coming from the other.

The difference between western medicine and acupuncture is that the orthodox western doctor uses these surface markings of inner diseases for diagnosis only, whereas the acupuncturist uses them for treatment too.

The Chinese classified the large number of acupuncture points into twelve main groups. All the points belonging to one of the twelve groups are joined by an imaginary line on the body's surface called a *meridian*. The twelve main meridians control the lung, large bowel, stomach, spleen, heart, small bowel, bladder, kidney, pericardium, 'triple warmer', gall-bladder and liver. All the acupuncture points along these meridians affect the organ named but not necessarily in the same way. The number of acupuncture points along any given meridian varies but, for example, the heart meridian has nine and the bladder

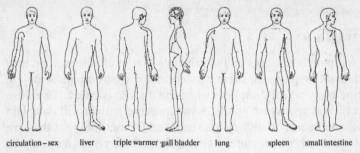

circulation – sex   liver   triple warmer ·gall bladder   lung   spleen   small intestine

The fourteen meridians

meridians sixty-seven on each side of the body. There are also two meridians placed centrally on the body, one on the front and the other down the back.

But the meridians aren't quite that simple because not only does stimulation of the points along their length affect the named internal organ but also the associated organs that developed with that organ embryologically. The main meridians also have branches that supply areas close to the main organs affected.

To the Chinese these meridians are an integral part of what makes us 'tick'. We in the West are very good on the medical plumbing but fall woefully short on most other things. The Chinese describe how the body's life forces – Chi – circulate in these meridians and then interpret all disease as a disturbance of these circulating life forces. Unfortunately, such a concept is difficult to grasp for hard-headed 'scientific' westerners because in acupuncture the physical and the metaphysical become somewhat blurred.

There is an accumulation of scientific evidence on how acupuncture works as we shall see but we in the West are still loath to accept it. There are several reasons for this. First, we can't believe that the Ancient Chinese could actually have anything to tell *us*; second, we can't yet pin down scientifically why it works; and third, acupuncturists themselves are not very helpful as they can only say *that* it works rather than why.

Modern pain research is shedding new light on how acupunc-

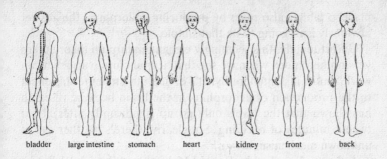

bladder   large intestine   stomach   heart   kidney   front   back

ture might work, though we still have no definite answers. Several authorities on pain and acupuncture claim, for example, that acupuncture meridians are no more real than geographical latitudes and longitudes on a map. Most of them agree though that acupuncture *points* certainly do exist. As one of the world's most eminent pain researchers, Professor Ronald Melzack, put it in a paper in the medical journal *Pain*: '. . . pressure at certain points is associated with particular pain patterns, and brief, intense stimulation of the points by needling sometimes produces prolonged pain relief'.

Just why this works is not known but exciting research in the US has shown that the brain produces natural pain-relieving substances, called endorphins, in response to acupuncture. Heroin addicts have lower than normal endorphin levels in their spinal fluid and this may give a clue to the success of acupuncture in the treatment of such addicts. Several practitioners in the UK, USA and Hong Kong claim some degree of success in the treatment of addicts with acupuncture using a kind of permanent stimulation acupuncture, achieved by inserting a staple in the person's earlobe. Another interesting finding is that the anti-narcotic drug, naloxone, not only reverses the effects of morphine, heroin and similar drugs but also blocks the analgesic action of acupuncture – thus proving that acupuncture and the most powerful pain killers known to Man are acting at the same brain receptors. But given that a fair percentage of people taking placebo tablets also react by producing endorphins, the answer obviously isn't going to be that simple.

Unfortunately, this seemingly elegant endorphin theory takes yet another knock when we see that acupuncture pain relief can work almost instantaneously. It's difficult to attribute this effect to the production of endorphins in the brain because research has shown that the levels only go up significantly after about twenty minutes of needling. So, clearly, there's another as yet unknown mechanism at work.

A theory described by Ronald Melzack and Patrick Wall, two of the world's most distinguished pain researchers, in 1965, might help provide some answers. They proposed the existence of a kind of 'gate' at every level in the spinal cord. This gate acts in such a way as to remain closed and so allow no pain stimuli to reach the brain. The theory is a highly complex one which is being modified all the time as knowledge expands but explained simply, it is roughly this. The gate in the spinal cord is constantly being bombarded by two kinds of stimuli, some trying to open it and others trying to close it. The balance is normally in favour of those trying to close the gate and hence we feel no pain most of the time. The gate can be influenced to open or close from above (by mental or psychological factors) or from outside (by painful stimuli) and both act in conjunction to control the degree to which the gate opens. The gate can be closed from above so that the person feels no pain even when he is subjected to a painful stimulus (this could explain how hypnosis blocks pain) and sometimes the gate can be opened from above to produce pain when there really is none (a condition known as psychogenic pain).

Acupuncture may well act in such a way as to close the gate in the spinal cord by stimulating 'shut-the-gate' or inhibitory pain pathways and this could explain why acupuncture has immediately perceivable results and later effects. The former are probably mediated via 'nervous' pathways (not along nerves as we know them in the anatomical sense but possibly along energy-conducting pathways that have no anatomical reality but simply create themselves transitorily as minute changes in the body's natural electrical fields) and the latter by chemical mediators in the brain (endorphins).

Having now seen how difficult it is to explain why acupuncture works, let's see how it's done.

How does it work?

It's fair to say that nobody knows – at least not in terms that can be understood by us in the West. But work it certainly does. Over the years acupuncture has been explained away as some kind of hypnosis. The fact that about 20 per cent of people don't respond to acupuncture (more in the West than in the East) seems to confirm this hypothesis but when one sees animals successfully treated, the hypnotic element seems to pale to insignificance. Acupuncture also works on completely anaesthetized patients. The most convincing evidence that acupuncture isn't a hypnotic phenomenon though is seen from studies of people who know what the results should be when they receive acupuncture treatment. They can tell the acupuncturist if he has placed the needle incorrectly by as little as one tenth of an inch. When the therapist replaces the needle, the patient then confirms the desired result. This could hardly be hypnosis.

In the early nineteenth century, the English physician Henry Head found that certain diseases of the internal organs were associated with excessive sensitivity at particular places on the skin. Each area of the body is served by a segment of the spinal cord which links a certain group of internal organs with specific areas of the body surface as explained above.

A fascinating case shows how complex this whole subject is. A Japanese doctor, Dr Nagahama, practising at a top Japanese university, was treating a patient who had been struck by lightning and had survived. The patient had extreme sensitivity of his skin as a result and was able to describe pathways (quite unknown to him) on his body that seemed to be stimulated when the doctor inserted the needle in an acupuncture point. The pathways the patient described were acupuncture meridians and *not* nervous pathways! Dr Nagahama then went on to find that the speed of transmission along these meridians was entirely different from that along nerves (about ten times slower) and also confirmed that there were interconnections between meridians as the Chinese had claimed for centuries.

In 1934, Dr George Crile, founder of the Cleveland Clinic, postulated that each human cell generated its own little electric current and so acted as a tiny battery but like so many real pioneers he was ridiculed in his own lifetime. Today, we know that he was right and studies of acupuncture points show that they have extraordinary electrical properties. The points can be distinguished electrically from surrounding skin and also differ electrically one from another. The Russians have developed an electronic machine called a tobiscope which flashes whenever it passes over an acupuncture point. A bright flash is said to show a healthy acupuncture point – a dull flash, potential or actual disease.

As yet we simply can't be sure about how the body's electrical fields (the life force or Chi of Chinese traditional medicine) function but we can be sure that they are there. It's interesting to note that the electrical potential of acupuncture points can be altered by the emotions too, so perhaps the patient's mental attitude *can* alter the outcome of acupuncture. A Far Eastern practitioner assures me that he gets measurably worse results in the West compared with the East and that this is probably caused by the entirely different frame of mind of people in the East. Hypnosis can also bring about changes in electrical potential at acupuncture points as can auto-suggestion and autogenic training, so the internal organs of the body seem to be controllable to some degree by higher brain centres and possibly through acupuncture meridians.

But to explain traditional Chinese medicine in such a typically reductionist western way is to debase it. The Chinese talk of the Chi – or body energy – circulating in our meridians twenty-five times a day and twenty-five times a night. They describe the interplay of yin and yang which are the very force of all life to the Chinese. Yin and yang are much more than our western concept of opposites (good and evil; hot and cold etc.) and rule the whole universe. Organs of the body are yin (solid ones) or yang (hollow ones) and the maintenance of health is centred around the balance of yin and yang within the body.

Ancient Chinese medicine also links the weather and the five main elements of wood, water, fire, metal and earth to health and disease. Every organ is linked with these five elements and also with yin and yang so that if, for example, the liver (wood) is stimulated, the heart (fire) will also be stimulated while the spleen (earth) will be sedated. Such seemingly nonsensical linkages can indeed be explained using modern neurophysiological knowledge. All this tends to prove what a few enlightened western doctors are beginning to realize – that you should not treat any one body organ in isolation. The organs have an interplay which we find difficult to explain with our restricted knowledge of anatomy but with which the Chinese are completely familiar. The trouble is that when someone starts linking the state of the weather and the cosmos with the way in which our spleen functions, he tends to be labelled a crank until proven otherwise. The Chinese have many of the answers but it'll be a long time before we can explain their mysteries in terms that western science can cope with.

Another amazing part of Chinese medicine and an integral part of acupuncture is pulse diagnosis. In fact it is the basis of traditional Chinese diagnosis. It is so sensitive a diagnostic method that it can tell of past illnesses so accurately that the doctor can regale a patient with his medical history. Pulse diagnosis can even warn of future ailments.

Pulse diagnosis seems like magic to those who can't do it but just as the working of a transistor seems like magic until it's explained, so, too, pulse diagnosis can be understood.

A traditional acupuncturist will be able to tell the state of the energy in the meridians by studying the patient's radial artery pulse at the wrist. There may be up to fourteen different sorts of pulse to be felt over the one artery at each wrist, but many acupuncturists think that five or six pulses are all they can hope to locate in practice. A Japanese electronics engineer has made an apparatus which, he claims, can differentiate between thirteen pulses at the wrist. The variables which he measures in the arteries are fullness, hardness, quietness and under- or overactivity. A highly experienced practitioner can diagnose hundreds of different conditions by feeling the pulse. The pulse at the wrist is also of diagnostic use to the western physician but by and large his interpretation is very much more restricted.

Pulse diagnosis is enormously skilful because, apart from actually having to distinguish all the possible pulses that can be felt, the acupuncturist also has to interpret the possibilities within any one area. For example, disturbances of the 'liver' pulse can be caused by at least nine 'livery' complaints from piles and biliousness to migraine and certain types of asthma.

Once the diagnosis has been made either from the pulse or by the study of the acupuncture points, how is acupuncture done?

How is it done?

There is only one skill in acupuncture – knowing where to stimulate the skin to achieve the desired result.

Usually the acupuncture points are stimulated with a needle but other methods of stimulation are widely practised. Moxibustion involves their stimulation with burning moxa (*Artemisia japonica*). Shiatsu stimulates them with the finger tips (see page 298) and true acupuncturists use a variety of stimuli including massage, electrical stimuli, mechanical vibrators, heat and magnetic oscillators. Most acupuncturists claim best results with needle stimulation.

The needles are usually made of a silver alloy or stainless steel. This renders them strong yet sterilizable and easy to keep sharp. Traditional Chinese textbooks describe some fifty different ways of inserting the needle but generally there are only six major things that govern the effectiveness of the stimulus once the needle is in the right spot:

1. The bore of the needle
2. The amount it is moved about
3. The depth to which it penetrates
4. The sharpness of the needle
5. The length of time the needle is left in place
6. The number of times the treatment is repeated.

Once the relevant acupuncture point has been located, the needle or needles are inserted and left there for any time from a few seconds to a few minutes. Some practitioners rotate the needles between their fingertips so as to stimulate the acupuncture point more vigorously while others simply insert the needle and remove it. Some acupuncturists claim to get better results by vibrating the needle electrically but this is open to debate.

A patient undergoing acupuncture treatment usually feels no pain. The public is somewhat horrified by the thought of needles being inserted vigorously to a great depth and are naturally apprehensive. Most acupuncturists do not cause pain and only insert the needles, which are extremely fine and sharp, a few millimetres into the skin. A greater stimulus does not necessarily mean a greater effect, so there is no virtue in acupuncture being painful. Treatments are usually carried out once or twice a week for chronic diseases and more often for acute ones.

Some people feel relief at once, within seconds, and some over several days. Certain patients need four or five treatments before any improvement is noticed, others describe a sense of lightness or buoyancy after a treatment and yet others a feeling of great relaxation. Occasionally an adverse reaction occurs before improvement starts which may alarm the patient if he isn't warned in advance. In about 20 per cent of people and in certain disease processes no result occurs at all.

What diseases respond best?

Theoretically any reversible disease can be cured with acupuncture and this is not far from reality in expert hands. A French physician, Dr J. Mauries, has treated 108 different ailments exclusively with acupuncture under the watchful eye of two other doctors. Numerous other series of cases abound the world over, especially in China.

The only proviso to be made is that the disease process must be caused by altered physiology. There is no point in using acupuncture to get rid of a kidney stone or advanced arthritis. The conditions that respond best of all are the short term dysfunctions of physiological processes such as headaches, acute lung disease, acute rheumatic conditions, menstrual, digestive and 'nervous' problems. So it's fair to say that acupuncture really only works for diseases which are potentially reversible and most acupuncturists won't waste time treating disease by acupuncture if orthodox medicine does the job well. For instance, if you've got pneumonia there's no point sticking needles in anywhere. A course of antibiotics is what's needed.

In China, it's rather different. A study in the Department of Surgery at Chung Shan Medical College, Canton, looked at thirty-six cases of acute appendicitis, ten of appendix abscess and three of perforated appendix with peritonitis. They were all treated with acupuncture (ten were also treated with Chinese herbs). Good results were obtained in all the cases without recourse to surgery, antibiotics or any of the procedures we in the West would have considered essential. Thirty of the thirty-six acute appendicitis cases were out of hospital within eight days.

In another study in Britain an acupuncturist treated forty consecutive patients with headaches that had baffled at least two other doctors previously. (Usually they had been seen by their general practitioner and a specialist before reaching him.) Eighty per cent were 'cured' or showed 'considerable improvement' and only three showed no improvement at all. This is remarkable by any standards and certainly can't be matched by modern western medicine.

To many of us in the West, though, acupuncture is synonymous with pain relief or alternatively with analgesia for operations. There's no doubt that it does work in relieving longstanding intractable pain as is borne out by many papers in the medical journals and there are many reports by western experts of the use of acupuncture in Chinese operating theatres. On his return from a trip to China Professor E. Gray Dimond, a world renowned American heart specialist, described having watched ten operations carried out under acupuncture analgesia. He told of seeing a Chinese surgeon with TB of the lung undergoing a surgical removal of his lung entirely under acupuncture – the needle being inserted into his left arm. 'The thorax gaped wide open. I could see his heart beating, and all the time the man was chatting cheerfully and quite coherently. When the procedure was about half-way finished the patient declared that he was hungry; the surgeons called a pause and gave him a jar of stewed fruit to eat.'

An Austrian surgeon, Dr Johannes Bischko, an acupuncturist of twenty years' standing, also witnessed such operations in China in 1972 and showed his films on German television. They showed a Caesarean section, the removal of a benign tumour, a dental extraction and the removal of part of a patient's lung. All the patients were conscious; none received any other medication; the needles were vibrated manually or electrically and some of the patients ate something during the procedure. This is all very well in China but similar experiences in the West are hard to come by. This is mainly because in China the patients are chosen very carefully and then subjected to a dummy run before the operation to see if they'll be suitable. The vast majority of Chinese have their operations carried out under chemical anaesthesia.

There have been at least 600,000 operations carried out in China under acupuncture analgesia since 1958 but research shows that it works only on a certain proportion of susceptible individuals. Faith and enthusiasm play an enormous part in its efficacy as an analgesic as was shown in a paper in the *British Journal of Anaesthesia*. In only 10 per cent of the people studied in the UK was there enough pain insensitivity to be able to carry out an operation. A further 65 per cent had a mild loss of pain sensations but certainly not enough for surgery. The author of the paper, a leading acupuncturist, suggested that this 10 per cent of successful patients are the 'strong reactors' who react powerfully to drugs as well as to acupuncture.

This same author now thinks that he was generous in allowing that 10 per cent of patients were anaesthetized by acupuncture. 'The level is really much more like 5 per cent,' he says ruefully. 'I'm afraid these people must be very strong reactors. In China they select their cases for anaesthesia very carefully and test them first to see if they'll come up to scratch on the day.'

After all, less than one million operations in such an enormous population over a period of twenty years doesn't mean that acupuncture is being used for everybody.

'A few doctors combine chemical anaesthesia with acupuncture in West Germany and think it works in many patients,' the acupuncturist continues. 'I've shown anaesthetist colleagues of mine the amount of drugs involved in these cases and they think that acupuncture contributes the effect of about two aspirins to the level of pain relief!'

Naturally this medical acupuncturist wishes these findings *weren't* true. After all, the popular press would have us believe that simple, safe anaesthetics with acupuncture are there for the asking, but this seems far from the truth today.

In spite of its shortcomings in the operating theatre, acupuncture still has much to offer in other fields, so why is it still on the fringe of medicine in the West? Is it just because we are slow to change and adopt new ideas?

According to a survey done by *Which* (the magazine of the Consumers' Association in Britain) most people who go to acupuncturists are the hopeless cases that orthodox medicine can't cure – yet 70 per cent of them improve. This is remarkable by any standards.

'The amazing thing to me is that people tell me it's all in the mind – that I have some sort of placebo effect,' says one practitioner, 'but frankly I don't mind. After all, I get excellent results whatever the explanation and they can't seriously suggest that I as an acupuncturist have any better a placebo effect than say a doctor in an impressive university medical school. Surely if someone thinks he is going to be cured, it's there that it's going to happen. They've got a head start on me when it comes to placebo effect!'

Acupuncture is still a minority art in the West. There are probably only about forty doctors practising it in the UK of whom only about four are full time acupuncturists. The rest are general practitioners who use acupuncture for say 20 per cent of their day.

In China today 500,000 doctors practise acupuncture and there are another 30,000 practitioners in Japan. In France and Germany it is used widely in hospitals and is available under their national health care systems. In Russia it is part of the curriculum in half a dozen universities and there are now well over 1,000 practitioners overall. In the whole of Europe there are probably more than 5,000 acupuncturists.

Most of the medically qualified acupuncturists feel that a medical degree is essential to practise safely. This seems very sensible because making the right diagnosis is an essential starting point and most lay practitioners simply can't know what they're treating. The danger will always be that a lay acupuncturist will be quite capable of treating things that are well defined but won't know enough medicine to recognize when his therapy isn't working because the underlying condition isn't in fact treatable.

It's in the twilight world of symptoms without frank disease that acupuncture works so well. The sobering fact is that very few diseases can be cured by western medicine mainly because by the time we recognize them they've taken a strong foothold and all we can do is use surgery or drugs to halt their progress.

Acupuncture can be used to pick up illness before this stage with a better chance of cure. After all, the Chinese doctor was traditionally only paid his fee when his patient was well. I suspect there'd be an enormous change in the pattern of health care in the West if we adopted this practice here!

The Alexander Technique

Definition

A technique to which the late Mr F. Matthias Alexander gave his name. It has been described as a method of posture training but it goes far beyond this simple concept and should be thought of as being more a technique by which mind and body are harmonized.

Background

F. Matthias Alexander was born in Tasmania in 1869 and became a reciter of poetry and humorous pieces. It was as a result of habitually losing his voice that he started to take more notice of his own body, its movements and balance. By studying himself in front of a mirror while reciting, he became aware that he was using his body wrongly. He noticed that every time he started to recite he pulled his head back and tightened his throat. Although such a seemingly strange posture felt normal to him he reasoned that it would be sensible to remedy it and so practised until he could recite properly without producing these strange movements and tensions. His voice improved and he no longer lost it when reciting.

Alexander trained himself to breathe and hold himself better and to pay a lot more attention to posture generally and soon felt much healthier and altogether more self-confident. He found himself encouraging and teaching others to do what he had found valuable and the good results spoke for themselves. He then created a system, based entirely on meticulous observation of himself and others, which encouraged people to unlearn the harmful or simply unhelpful habitual movements of their every-day lives, so freeing them of strange, 'unnatural' postures and movements. He found that the worst offenders used their bodies badly when changing from sitting to standing or lying to sitting, often by throwing their heads backwards.

After ten years of teaching in Australia and New Zealand, Alexander went to London in 1904. His work and ideas slowly gained recognition and between 1914 and 1918, and 1940 and 1943 he worked in New York. He left his younger brother, A. R. Alexander, to develop his methods in the USA. His book *The Use of Self* was published in 1932 and from then on his teachings spread widely throughout the western world. He died in 1955 aged eighty-seven and left a small number of teachers to carry on his work. Today there are training schools all over the world but the main ones are in London. There is a Society of Teachers of the Alexander Technique with major schools in Israel, Zürich,

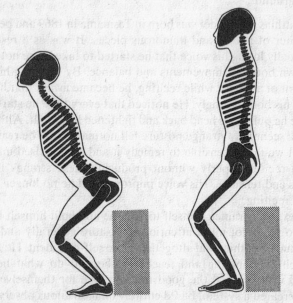

The incorrect (left) and correct (right) way of sitting down

London, San Francisco, Chicago and The Hague but the majority of teachers of the technique are still to be found in and around London.

How is it done?

Unlike many alternative medical therapies, the Alexander technique is not simply a 'treatment' in which someone does something to someone else. Rather it is a self re-education process, encouraged and led by an expert. When you think about it, even the most simple daily movements, such as getting up and opening a door, are highly complex and involve the careful balancing of many muscle groups. Alexander teachers help the individual rediscover his basic, natural posture and movement patterns by liberating the body from learned, superimposed ones. In this way neuro-muscular co-ordination is improved generally. This means that at first as the old, 'wrong' movements and postures are corrected the new ones feel strange but soon these feel right with all the attendant improvements on the mind and body. There are no exercises as such to be done by the Alexander student but it may take up to a year of practice in one's daily life to get the full benefit.

By the time most of us have reached adult life we will have acquired harmful postural habits which induce mental and physical tension. Alexander's principle is a new way of organizing oneself and it's a serious business. Just as with any other useful therapy the first stage is to make some sort of diagnosis. The Alexander teacher (and I say teacher because the vast majority are not doctors) does this by establishing which forms of misuse and bad posture are present in the pupil.

The pupil is asked to lie on a flat, firm surface at couch height. He is then encouraged to 'inhibit' or prevent any seemingly normal reflex movements as the teacher handles and moves his body. Slowly the pupil learns a whole new vocabulary of body movement as the teacher moves various parts of the body to relieve tension and adjust posture. The pupil learns to associate

certain groups of words and instructions with the correct position
in which the teacher places him and it is this that he continues
on his own when his teacher is not there. Clearly the pupil has
to be completely involved in the process which may require eight
forty-five minute sessions over many weeks and perhaps further
follow-up visits. Over this period the pupil learns not only to
inhibit bad movements, tensions and postures, but positively to
'direct' his body to do the right thing. The idea is that after such
re-education much of this learning becomes second nature,
although most people find that conscious attention to it will be
needed.

The Alexander technique is in no way cranky or way-out; at
least, in the best hands it isn't. All Alexander said in essence was
that for each of us there is an optimum posture and movement

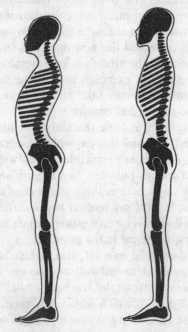

The incorrect (left) and correct (right) way of standing

pattern which suits us best. The techniques used by Alexander teachers simply help the pupil return to this optimal resting state without tension after the normal movements of everyday life. After all, we all have to stretch for things, and many of us sit badly at office desks, hunch over the wheel in our cars and go to sleep in awkward postures in front of the television. The trouble is that for the non-Alexander trained person these bad habits become ingrained and produce physical ill health.

How does it work?

The Alexander technique is not orthodox but it is not inconsistent with accepted principles of physiology and psychology either. It has nothing in common with the many techniques of auto-suggestion, relaxation, transcendental meditation or other methods of mind control. Basically the method teaches a person to discriminate between movement and posture cues in such a way as to enable him to eliminate the parts of a learned response pattern that interfere with optimal performance or function of the body. To understand this better, let's look at some basic facts about Man and his ancestors.

A four-legged animal has its head in front of its body and its neck muscles are constantly acting to hold its head up against gravity. The forward movement of the head pulls on the spine and the head's movement 'leads' the body into its various activities.

The same basic mechanism applies in Man. As we start a body movement we move our heads in the direction we intend to take and these tiny movements are recorded by minute variations in the lengths of the muscle fibres in the neck muscles. If we consider how a baby learns to walk we see that the first stage involves the raising of its head against gravity. Once head control is achieved the body follows and after a time he has perfect head control and is soon walking. Babies and young children have easy, unimpaired head control. As the child gets older though he becomes subject to anxiety and stressful and posturally unnatural situations which can cause abnormal contractions of the spinal and neck muscles, so shortening the neck a fraction.

In addition to the frankly stressful conditions in which we live, many people are lazy about the way they walk, sit and hold themselves and over many years their bodies become rebalanced to cope with their slouching, rounded shoulders, rounded backs and drooping heads. This slouching posture alters the expansion capabilities of the chest and so impairs breathing.

Professor Frank Pierce Jones in Massachusetts, not content with what he knew to be the results of the Alexander Method that he had seen in his own and other people's lives, set about explaining all this in high-powered scientific terms that would be acceptable to sceptics. Much of Alexander's original work was written in philosophical rather than scientific language and this did nothing to recommend it to a scientific and technological society. It is partly because of this difficulty that the method has not enjoyed greater popularity, especially among the medical profession.

The Alexander technique lends itself to experimentation very well, mainly because a skilled teacher can change posture in a subject very quickly. The subjects in Pierce Jones's experiment were asked to grade the effort required to maintain three different types of posture. The first was the person's usual relaxed (often slouching) posture; the second was his usual erect posture (his 'best' posture); and the third was an experimental posture (as guided by Alexander principles). All the subjects found that they needed more effort to maintain their 'best' posture than they did to maintain the Alexander posture and that the Alexander posture was more effortless even than their usual 'slouched' posture. These findings were all subsequently confirmed using electromyography to measure actual electrical potentials in the muscles of the neck.

The subjects described their Alexander-trained movements as 'smoother, easier and lighter' compared with their normal ones and Pierce Jones set out to confirm this by using slow motion films. He found that the subjects' Alexander trained movements were carried out faster than their original movements and concluded that the power provided by the muscles must have been proportionately greater, since the end position obtained was the same whether the subjects were using the Alexander method or not.

Pierce Jones's and other people's work supports the following hypotheses about the Alexander principle:

1. The basic postural reflexes of the body are integrated with other reflex systems (which comes as no news to practitioners of yoga, see page 308).

2. Under civilized conditions these reflexes are partly inhibited by habitual, learned responses which disturb the relationship between the head, neck and trunk.

3. Once this inhibition is drawn to the attention of the person, he can be taught to prevent it with general improvement of body function.

But probably the best experimental work has been carried out by an Englishman, Dr W. Barlow (who is married to Alexander's niece). He knew Alexander personally and has carried out numerous studies on this subject over the last quarter of a century. Dr Barlow is a physician in a big London hospital and sees patients treated by all the conventional means that modern medicine has to offer. Yet he finds that the Alexander technique has much more to offer in many cases. He has yet to find a case of backache – that scourge of western man – that he cannot help with the aid of the technique and also gets excellent results with migraine, depressions and neuroses of all kinds.

His major study of the technique involved the minute anthropometric measurement of fifty Royal College of Music students in London. He subjected them all to Alexander training and took further measurements after six months. Forty-nine of them were up to 1¾ inches taller and had greatly improved in terms of musicianship. In another study he examined the effects of the Alexander technique on students at the Central School of Speech and Drama in London. The teachers at the School did all they could to help these students improve their posture, breathing and so on using their usual training techniques, but after one year all were measurably worse off. The Alexander technique subsequently improved them all.

What is it used for?

Because the Alexander method aims at redressing postural balance, it is of most value to actors, musicians and dancers, who greatly benefit from the training. However, because it increases a person's sense of well-being and even improves frankly unwell people on occasions, it is becoming increasingly popular as a kind of medical therapy. It should be stressed that it is not primarily a way of curing specific ailments although a few doctors use it as an addition to their armamentarium of treatments.

The Alexander technique has been useful to people with specific postural problems, breathing troubles and speech defects. Alexander himself never meant his method to become a type of curative medical therapy but rather to be a self-help method.

People often ask whether it has anything to do with meditation, yoga or similar practices. The answer is that it depends very much on the individual. Some people combine yoga or Zen Buddhism with the Alexander technique but the technique itself is not inherently spiritual. One of the world's leading experts was quite happy to call it a sort of 'super physiotherapy with additional benefits'. In the right hands though it can go way beyond whatever the best physiotherapy has to offer.

Does it work?

Quite simply the answer is 'yes'. Like almost any treatment that involves the individual attention of a skilled and sympathetic person for long periods of time, the Alexander technique undoubtedly works as a kind of supportive psychotherapy for many people. One leading practitioner tells how his patients slowly unwind mentally as well as physically and gradually the real cause of their problems emerges, such as a difficult inter-personal relationship or some other domestic or work upset. But Alexander has more to offer than this as can be seen in people who have had very little verbal contact with their teacher. Quite how it works is a matter that is likely to be debated for years but most of us in western medicine have completely overlooked the importance of correct posture in the head and neck and the way that information is fed back from muscles there to many parts of the brain. This may seem a very strange concept at first but can be better understood if we consider how muscles receive their nerve inputs.

The lengthening (or shortening) of muscles is not simply related to the 'all or nothing' switching on or off of their nerve supply. There are two systems of nerves in muscles that we know about today – indeed until fairly recently we only knew about the first. This first system works by contracting and shortening muscle fibres. When this system stops 'firing', the muscle relaxes. The second system is a collection of nerves that don't actually go to the muscles that we can feel in our bodies but to masses of microscopic bundles called muscle spindles. These are buried deep in the muscles, lie lengthways in between the muscle fibres and are involved in muscle lengthening rather than contraction.

Muscle spindles have their own internal muscles which feed information about their state of contraction or relaxation back to the brain. These spindles are the fine tuning system of our muscles and also prevent excessive contraction and relaxation of muscles during activity. They therefore act as a sort of shock absorber or damper in a highly complex way. It can be shown that over-shortening of a muscle (such as is seen in certain bad postures and habits) causes the muscle spindles to go 'dead' so that there is no feedback from them to the brain. This might not seem very important but is in reality because the brain connec-tions of all the millions of muscle spindles from all over our bodies interact with all kinds of higher centres that play a vital part in our awareness of what's happening around us. Suffice it to say that powerful pain-killers like morphine act by dulling or temporarily inactivating this very same area of the brain that is 'turned off' when our muscle spindles cease to function.

When we understand all this it then makes a lot of sense to talk of people feeling altogether fitter and healthier simply by getting them to breathe properly (and more deeply) because by doing so they are activating muscle spindles that have been dormant for some time. (For more details of this kind of phenomenon, see page 311.)

But for all this detailed knowledge we still don't know why so many conditions from back pain, arthritis and breathing disorders to stress diseases are helped by the Alexander technique. Like so many areas of fringe medicine, the technique deserves far more serious research than it has so far enjoyed. It shouldn't be difficult to convince most western doctors that there's something in it – the patients (pupils) speak for themselves and the work of Barlow and others like him cannot easily be dismissed or ignored. If only because the Alexander technique is a safe, self-help technique that can save any health care system a fortune, it deserves far greater popularity and attention.

Anthroposophical Medicine

Definition

An extension of medical thinking and practice based on and inspired by the work and teaching of Rudolf Steiner.

Background

Rudolf Steiner (1861–1925) was the son of a minor Austrian railway official. As a very young boy, he already realized that he had unusual powers of perception. These powers eventually led him into many different fields of study and to his achievements being acclaimed by experts in these fields. Although many people call Steiner a mystic, he always regarded himself as a spiritual scientist.

Steiner was educated at the Vienna Technical University, where he soon became interested in philosophy and attended university courses on the subject. He also taught himself the classics and was keenly interested in literature and the arts. This combination of science and the arts led him to Goethe and at the age of twenty-three he was invited to edit Goethe's scientific works. During this time he laid the foundations for what he later called Anthroposophy. He obtained a Ph.D. at Rostock University and came to be recognized as the leading authority on Goethe's scientific works.

In 1897 he became a professional literary editor in Berlin. Until that time his lectures and writings had been clothed in language in which nothing direct was said about perceptions of spiritual beings and spiritual worlds. He now began to feel an increasing urgency to speak more openly, both out of a personal need and also in response to the growing tendency inherent in nineteenth-century science to imprison man in a consciousness limited to material entities and mechanical processes. This meant that he had to adopt a different approach and a different vocabulary to describe the world as he saw it. This predictably amazed, baffled and alienated many people, but he found sympathetic audience among members of the Theosophical Society, within which he worked as a writer, lecturer and teacher until 1912. His subjects included the theory and practice of developing spiritual perception. He believed that this insight into the spiritual world was potentially accessible to everybody. However, he warned against the adoption of techniques designed to produce quick results in terms of altered states of consciousness which were not accompanied by an equivalent degree of moral development.

Steiner always tried to express himself in a rational and scientific way, appealing to common sense rather than belief in authority. Even before his association with the Theosophical Society, Steiner had come to see the incarnation of Christ as a unique event and a spiritual turning point for the life of the earth and for mankind. Although Steiner had previously written some sharp criticisms of doctrinal and organized Christianity, his 'conversion' was a determining factor for the rest of his life. When in 1912 a young Indian boy was proclaimed by some leading members of the Theosophical movement to be a new incarnation of Christ, Steiner refused to go along with this and was excluded from the Theosophical Society. In 1913 he founded the Anthroposophical Society. (The word *anthroposophy* comes from the Greek *anthropos* – man, and *sophia* – wisdom.)

The headquarters of the Anthroposophical Society were established in Dornach near Basle, Switzerland. A suitable building was designed by Steiner personally. This was no small task as the building consisted of two intersecting domes, one of which was larger than the dome of St Paul's in London. Although he had received no formal architectural training he was able to work out all the mathematical details for the intersection of the two domes of unequal size, much to the amazement of leading architects of the day who had said it couldn't be done. The building, constructed entirely of wood, marked the beginning of a new development in architecture. Steiner also inspired and directed the painting and carving work in the interior. The building was, unfortunately, destroyed by fire in 1923 but Steiner designed a replacement which was one of the first buildings in the world to be made entirely of reinforced concrete.

Over the years this incredible genius of a man attracted all kinds of people who wanted to find out what his views of the world could offer them in their particular fields of work. He attracted artists, teachers of normal and backward children, farmers, actors, church ministers, scientists and doctors, all eager to learn. Steiner lectured to such people throughout his life and astounded experts in their fields with his perception and deep knowledge of their subjects – subjects in which he had no formal qualifications. Just before his death he was lecturing on mathematics, theology, philosophy, science, astronomy, drama, education, social science, economics and many other topics besides medicine.

Steiner was not a doctor of medicine nor did he intend to create a special branch of medicine, yet his spiritual insight has led thousands of doctors to change their ways of thinking and practice. The founding of hospitals, mostly in Germany and Switzerland, devoted to his ideas means that hundreds of thousands of people have been treated according to his medical indications.

What is it?

To get a clearer idea of what anthroposophical medicine is, we need to look at Steiner's objections to standard medical philosophy and practice and then see how he overcame them.

In the scientific medical world, all our attempts at understanding the human body are centred around 'reductionism'. We firmly believe that by reducing everything far enough we will one day learn all the secrets of life and therefore be able to cure everything. Even psychological diseases and disturbances, it is argued, will eventually be explicable in terms of brain cellular biochemistry.

Although such a view of Man and his ailments has yielded good results in certain fields, it's becoming apparent that such an approach has its shortcomings. It is now doubted whether the genetic material we all carry could possibly contain enough information to describe the structure and control processes of the body, let alone all the intermediary forms of the body as it develops. The development of the embryo is by no means understood and the controlling 'forces' or memories in the genetic material seem insufficient to explain everything we observe. Don't forget that in the adult too, cells are constantly being destroyed and rebuilt. The overall form of our bodies remains constant but the substance of the form is changing every moment of our lives. It has been calculated that our bodies are completely renewed about every seven years. In other words all the atoms that make up our physical framework will have been exchanged for others over a seven year period. This means that living organisms (of which we happen to be one of the most complicated) have a complexity involving time as well as space. We have no real idea how this is governed – and biochemistry doesn't seem to provide the answer.

Steiner claimed that if we limit our science of man only to those things that can be perceived by the physical senses, then we miss out on a whole dimension of Man, his life and his illnesses. Professor D. W. Smithers (Professor of Radiotherapy at the University of London) also found the reductionist ideas of medicine too restricting when studying the cancer patient. He maintained that it was as impossible to deduce the form of the human body from a study of the properties of his individual cells as it would be to deduce the rules of a game of billiards from the study of the properties of individual billiard balls.

Steiner described how formative processes work, how they work in different parts of the body and how they work in health and disease. He laid great stress on the fact that man is not only much more highly developed than animals and plants but that he has another dimension altogether, Steiner felt that this inner life of Man, his sense of self-identity, set him apart from all other living things.

All this led Steiner to describe a fourfold picture of Man. Man, he said, has a physical body (the basic 'plumbing'); he has another body that is living and full of creative forces (the 'etheric' body); he also has an inner life of emotions and drives (what Steiner called the 'astral' body); and, lastly, he is conscious of himself as an 'I'. All these four interrelate and none is governed by the laws of the other.

This means that the anthroposophical doctor sees disease in a rather different way from most. To him disease is not simply a collection of signs and symptoms but is an expression of a malfunctioning of all four of Man's 'bodies'. Such an approach enables the anthroposophical doctor to piece together a kind of imaginative picture of the patient and so help him accordingly. This is very much in keeping with the current vogue in medicine that realizes that very many more 'diseases' arise in the mind than we ever thought before.

But not only does such a broad and spiritual approach help the doctor make a diagnosis and explain the disease – it also helps him treat the patient more adequately. Steiner put great importance on understanding the true nature of plants and thus their value as medicines. Plants not only concentrate certain minerals but, he maintained, collect other forces surrounding them from the cosmos.

With regard to therapy, Steiner accepted that homoeopathy was a serious medical discipline and foresaw the problems of harming people with large doses of drugs when he wrote: 'When they are taken into the body they are "foreign bodies causing disturbances and over loading, if the body is burdened with the forces contained in allopathic doses." '

As regards diet, Steiner said that meat eating leaves the job of digesting vegetable food to the vegetarian animals we eat. So, he reasoned, the meat eater doesn't maintain the ability to digest vegetable food as the vegetarian can and so doesn't derive the energies he should from the plant food he does eat. This means he has to contend with energies peculiar to the animals he eats. The energies for 'overcoming' plant food are there but if they're not used, they rebound into the organism and produce exhaustion and irritation. However, Steiner was not a complete vegetarian unlike many of the Eastern mystics who have advocated vegetarianism.

Steiner's unique contribution to modern psychology and physiology was his theory that not all the aspects of Man's psychological life are centred in the brain.

Steiner saw man as having three interrelated dynamic parts. The 'thinking' parts are found in the brain, nerves and sense organs, and control consciousness and thinking. The second part is centred in the chest and consists of the heart, lungs and major blood vessels. It is rhythmic and spreads awareness throughout the body. It balances out the first and third systems, whose activities otherwise frequently conflict.

The third system is that concerned with metabolism, reproduction and movement. It deals with the conversion of food to body substance and energy transformation and provides the physiological basis for life.

He then explained how plants have much the same threefold structure, only upside down. The root (like the brain) is isolated from external influences, yet controls everything. Roots when digested stimulate the 'nerve-sense' system, according to Steiner. The stem and the leaves carry the ebb and flow of water and salts and correspond to the rhythmic system of the heart and lungs in Man, while the flower and fruit are metabolically active, mediate between the plant and the cosmos and correspond to the instinct and movement systems in Man.

Because Steiner held that a person's emotional life was so important to his total health, he insisted that any physical treatment of the body should be backed up by treatment of the mind. To this end he devised physical and artistic therapies which develop the harmonious balance between mind and body so essential for health.

Eurythmy is an art of movement, based on original ideas of Rudolf Steiner, which 'expresses the gestures inherent in speech and music'. This has been developed in one direction as an art and in another as a therapy. In curative eurythmy certain gestures are used in a specific and exaggerated way to redress a particular imbalance in the human organism. It can be of special value in loosening what has been called the body's 'character armour', the habitual patterns of movement and posture that we tend to adopt in response to our environment and especially to stress. In this particular respect it can achieve a similar effect to that of the Alexander technique (see page 83).

As well as movement therapy, a kind of painting therapy has since been developed by Steiner's pupils, a therapy which is now used in a number of medical centres through continental Europe.

The meaning of illness

From an anthroposophical point of view, illness is not merely an evil to be eliminated at all costs. If worked with constructively, it can be the gateway to new possibilities in life. We can learn something about the way we are abusing ourselves mentally and physically and so alter our way of life. As many illnesses have their origin in an imbalance in the 'soul life' an illness can itself be a way of overcoming that imbalance. It is the task of the doctor to discover what is behind the illness and help the patient work *with* it. If in spite of all attempts to cure the illness and preserve life, the patient dies, this does not mean that all the effort has been in vain. According to anthroposophy, Man's life on earth is not limited to this one incarnation. As psychological problems can be manifest as illnesses in one life time, so do problems of the soul which have not been overcome in one life tend to be manifest as constitutional weaknesses, physical malformations or illnesses in the next life. Such handicaps can then help the person to overcome the original imbalance, or to develop a particular strength of soul for a future life, according to anthroposophical doctors.

This sort of thinking helps anthroposophical doctors to look at abnormalities in a positive way and has led to the foundation of many highly successful schools with international reputations for children in need of special care. There are well over 1,000 children in these special schools in Britain alone who are receiving what Steiner called 'curative education', and many thousands of other children have benefited from such special care on the continent of Europe.

What of the future?

Steiner was undoubtedly a genius and a man with tremendous spiritual vision. He did most of his work on anthroposophical medicine in the latter part of his life and by the time he died not many doctors had started to put his ideas into practice. Much of his writing was, and still is, difficult for the average doctor to understand because of its unconventional language and often poor translation from the German. This has meant that however valuable and thought-provoking many of his ideas might be, they are difficult for most of us to grasp.

In order to be an anthroposophical doctor, one first has to be a medical doctor and then start to learn all over again. It is almost impossible to become an anthroposophical doctor without establishing a fundamental relationship with anthroposophy itself. Out of this one can then begin to transform one's previously acquired medical knowledge, with the help of experienced anthroposophical medical practitioners, by reading Steiner's writings and lectures, by working on one's own inner development and by practising the kind of observation of man and nature first developed by Goethe. This is hard going for all but the real zealot and is another reason why an approach so much in tune with modern trends towards a wholistic approach to life hasn't caught on in the English-speaking world. Much of what Steiner said still remains to be proved by scientific methods and to many seems cranky but I am sure we will find that his extraordinary powers of perception and spiritual awareness will be vindicated as we discover at our slower pace that he was right about many things. Since his death, many of his teachings have been borne out by scientific research but the work of such a genius will take centuries to elucidate. For example, he told of the importance of fluoride to the teeth in the 1920s and was talking about lead poisoning from atmospheric lead long before it was thought to be a problem.

   Although Steiner's medical foresight was phenomenal, the greatest challenge of anthroposophical medicine is that the doctor practising it needs to cultivate his powers of spiritual awareness. Training oneself to this level of awareness and at the same time correlating one's spiritual perceptions with laboratory results and the findings of physical examination is a long process and will by definition only be achieved by relatively few who feel motivated to cultivate such powers of perception, while retaining a commitment to the scientific approach of Man and to nature. While many doctors are content to treat only the physical part of man, the really good doctor, whether he has heard of anthroposophy or not, is, according to anthroposophists, treating the fourfold being of Man, even if he is not aware of it himself.

Aromatherapy

Definition

A combination of body and face massage using essential oils extracted from plants. On one level it can be practised as a sophisticated form of herbal medicine (as some of the oils can be taken internally too) and on another it can simply be a relaxing beauty therapy.

Background

Most of us are aware that plants contain chemical substances of various kinds that can be extracted and used for the benefit of mankind. The contraceptive pill, derived from Mexican yams, is probably the best known and most widely used of these natural plant extracts in the West.

However, what most people don't know is that plant extracts have been used for centuries and have therefore stood the test of time, unlike modern drugs most of which have only been with us for fifty years or less.

Specifically, aromatherapy uses the *essences* from plants rather than the whole or even part of the plants themselves. The essence of a plant is made up of aromatic (smelly) oils that appear in the various parts of a given plant in differing amounts at various times of the day. They can occur in the roots (for example in calamus), the flowers (lavender), the leaves (rosemary), the bark (sandalwood), and even in the resin (myrrh). They are also found in the rind of some fruits.

These naturally occurring oils are thought to be the very 'personality' of the plant itself, and no two are alike. They may well be waste products of plant metabolism but nobody really knows. They are formed in different parts of the plant and then circulated so that in the evening the essence may be most concentrated in the flowers, for example, and in the morning in the leaves. The chemical and medicinal properties of an essence extracted from a particular part of a plant differ according to the part of the plant they come from. For example, essence extracted from the orange tree flower acts very differently in the human body compared with that extracted from orange rind.

In the plants themselves, essential oils act as pesticides, fungicides and bactericides and may also have some hormone-like properties.

Aromatic oils are widely used in modern society in foods, toiletries and pharmaceuticals. Lemon and orange are probably the most popular ones used in foods; cosmetics and toiletries draw widely on these substances too, while clove oil for toothache and eucalyptus inhalations are well known to any 'kitchen table' doctor. The oils are also widely found as components of tonics, hair oils, inhalants and many other patent medicines.

These essences occur only in the tiniest amounts in plants and so have to be carefully and painstakingly extracted, which makes them expensive. It takes 2,000 pounds of rose petals to produce one pound of rose oil and the tedious distillation processes involved in the extraction make the production of synthetic alternatives attractive at first sight. Unfortunately, it appears from research done by a leading French expert, Valnet, that exactly similar chemical substances reproduced in the laboratory *do not* have the same properties as the naturally occurring essences – so there is no alternative but to use the real thing.

In order to retain the properties of the essential oils the method of extraction employed is very important. If the essential oils have been obtained by distillation, their effect is not as remarkable as those obtained by enfleurage. This is a method of extraction carried out as follows: flowers or plants are spread out on filters which are then placed in a bowl of oil. The oil, after a period of time, absorbs the 'odoriferous molecules' of the plants, which are replaced frequently until the oil is completely saturated. The oil is then separated from the essence by distillation. The essences are then dissolved in cold, pressed vegetable oils. Alcohol is never used as it destroys the valuable properties of the essences.

The history of essences is long and distinguished. The Egyptians probably did most for aromatherapy (although they didn't call it this) thousands of years ago at about the same time as the Chinese were developing acupuncture. When Tutenkhamun's tomb was opened in 1922, many scent pots were found which showed that frankincense and myrrh were widely used by the rich of the day. Patients in ancient times knew only too well many of the powerful properties of essential oils. In fact, medicines and perfumes were interchangeable in ancient Egypt. The Greeks used plant oils to heal wounds and reduce inflammation and the Romans used them widely too.

In Britain it wasn't until the sixteenth century when a botanist, William Turner, started classifying plants in terms of their effects on the human body, that the subject became of any great interest. At first the 'Doctrine of Signatures' held sway. This stated that if a plant or some part of it had an appearance similar to a part of the body, then it was probably active on that part of the body but as a more 'scientific' approach to medicine became fashionable, this doctrine lost much of its popularity.

By the end of the eighteenth century, essential oils were widely used in medicine and a *Herbal* of 1722 listed thirteen as 'official' preparations.

Soon, though, herbs and essential oils were abandoned as chemistry flourished as a scientific discipline and more powerful and faster-acting substances could be made. Slowly but surely essences lost their place in pharmacopoeias and the whole subject became thought of as cranky and obscure.

This was very much the position when a Frenchman, Gattefossé, working in his laboratory early this century, burned his hand while conducting an experiment. He doused his hand in a dish of lavender oil that happened by chance to be nearby and was astonished at the speed with which the hand healed. He it was who coined the term aromatherapy in the first book on the subject published in 1928.

In 1938, a Frenchman, M. Goddissart, working in Los Angeles, was reporting excellent results in the treatment of skin cancer, gangrene and wound healing. Dr Valnet, also a Frenchman, used aromatherapy widely in the Second World War to heal wounds and help good scar healing and it was his work, published in 1964, that led to much of our current knowledge of the subject.

The last person in the chain of the development of this remarkable form of medicine is Mme Maury, a biochemist, who extended the subject to cosmetology and rejuvenation.

How does it work?

The essences extracted from plants are complex natural oils. They contain esters, alcohols, aldehydes, ketones and terpenes.

Nobody knows exactly how essences work in the body but there again we don't know how many drugs work and we still use them. Aspirin had been widely used for nearly seventy years before its mode of action was understood, yet it was and still is the most widely used medicine in the world, with fifteen million tablets being taken every day in the UK alone. Just as we know that aspirin works, so physicians and healers have known for centuries that aromatic oils have curative properties.

Essential oils can be taken internally, inhaled or massaged through the skin. We all know that certain culinary herbs affect digestion and we can easily understand that the inhalation of eucalyptus and other aromatic oils can be useful. But when it comes to substances being absorbed through the skin, most of us would draw the line. However, modern research is proving that much more passes through the skin than we ever thought possible and some of the best academic units in the world are looking at ways of getting drugs into people directly through the skin surface straight to the problem area. This research is already showing that some drugs can easily be absorbed through the skin from deposits of the drugs placed on the skin surface for long periods.

There are many learned papers written on the subject of substances passing through the skin and some drugs given as creams and ointments by today's doctors are well known to affect the body generally. Corticosteroid (steroid) cream, especially if applied under occlusive dressings, can cause a dangerous build up of steroids in the body. Research has also shown that drugs whose actions and activities are well known to us act differently when absorbed through the skin compared with their actions when taken orally. So this could mean that aromatic oils have effects that we cannot even guess at simply by looking at them as chemicals. Their mode of action is even more complex than this, though, because they're not single chemical entities but highly complex groups that probably interact with each other both on the skin and in the body.

But let's go back to the basic property of aromatic oils – their smell. Nobody really knows what 'smell' means. The concept of smelling is infinitely more complicated than most doctors and scientists ever thought. Smelly substances (and most of the essential oils are smelly in a very pleasant way) produce so-called *'odoriferous molecules'*. These are picked up by the nose and interpreted as a recognizable smell by specialized parts of the brain.

The art and science of perfumery is based on the fact that smells are sexually (or even simply pleasantly) appealing. There are cultural differences the world over but it's interesting to note how many similarities there are in what people separated by thousands of miles and years in time find attractive. The application of smells to the skin in this way may have more implications than the girl behind the cosmetic counter realizes. Is it possible, for example, that we can 'smell' with our skin as well as our noses? Some interesting Russian research has found that some people can (and others can be trained to) 'feel' colours. After a short training people can learn to distinguish colours very accurately with their fingertips whilst blindfolded. It is well known that under the influence of LSD people 'hear' tastes, 'smell' colours and so on, so perhaps 'smelling' through the skin surface is a faculty which we have all but lost in the process of evolution.

Aromatherapy uses neither animal oils nor mineral oils – all the oils used come from plants. The oils, once taken, are absorbed and are then dispersed throughout the body's extracellular fluids. According to Tisserand in his book on aromatherapy, some are taken up by specific body organs and others are distributed more generally. Why this happens we don't know but it may well be that by stimulating the local blood supply by massage, the oils are especially well absorbed by organs supplied by these blood vessels. As nerves too have a blood supply, this could explain how these oils can act on the nerves directly and so cause effects at a distance. When the oils have been taken (injected, inhaled or massaged through the skin), they are excreted mainly via the lungs and the urine but others are excreted after being changed in the body (just like many drugs). Some essences are too toxic to be used internally in the required dose. Dosage is important because some oils act differently in different concentrations. Oils of melissa and rosemary for example are sedative or stimulating depending upon the dose. Like any form of medicine, the therapeutic dosage has to be worked out once the diagnosis has been made.

There has not been nearly enough research into the effects of aromatic oils and how they work in the body but interest is beginning to grow as people become disenchanted with the side-effects of many of the powerful drugs produced today. Hopefully, modern research units will restart where other scientists in the past left off.

In 1963 a Japanese team found that fennel, peppermint, cardamom and other oils had an antispasmodic activity in the intestine of mice.

An Italian paper as long ago as 1925 showed that the amount of saliva produced by people whose tongues had been deadened to taste by blocking the taste nerves, depended greatly on whether the smell of the oils was pleasant or unpleasant. It's interesting to speculate that if these digestive glands (the salivary glands) can be affected in this way, others lower down the bowel may well be too.

Several essential oils are natural laxatives and act by mildly increasing the squeezing movement the bowel normally exerts on its contents. Many more, though, relax the bowel wall and reduce spasm.

In the cardiovascular system, the effects of aromatic oils are less dramatic. Calamus reduces blood pressure and some oils given orally help improve the peripheral circulation.

The antispasmodic effects of these oils are especially effective in the lungs. In 1970 a study showed that the expectorant action of lemon oil (given as a steam inhalation) was greatest at a level which couldn't be perceived by the sense of smell. The use of aromatic substances to increase mucus production by the lungs and so help bring up phlegm is well known to us all but, until this work, it was not known just how powerful these oils were. Subsequent experiments have shown that very low doses of the oils greatly increase mucus production in the lungs, so aiding the coughing up of troublesome phlegm in patients with chronic lung disease such as bronchitis.

Although most plant oils do not act as hormones in the plants they come from, many have hormonal properties in humans. The plant sarsaparilla contains the male sex hormone testosterone; hops, fennel and aniseed contain oestrogens; and *vitex agnus castus* contains progesterone-like substances. A few essences contain substances hormonally active in man but usually it's the whole plant that contains them. There is an enormous future in the isolation and extraction of many of these substances. The contraceptive pill is just one example of what can be achieved.

How is it done?

Aromatic oil therapy (aromatherapy) is not widely practised in the UK (where there is probably only a handful of true aromatherapists) but is fairly commonplace in France and on the continent of Europe generally. In the UK, liberal laws mean that anyone can call himself an aromatherapist and set up a practice to treat people. In France this is not the case and aromatherapists (along with other specialists in alternative medicine) can practise only under the watchful eye of a medically trained doctor. On the continent of Europe, aromatherapy is usually used as an integral part of some other alternative therapy such as osteopathy, acupuncture or radiesthesia, but in the UK it is practised more often alone as a treatment in its own right.

The starting point, as with any medical treatment, is the arrival at some sort of diagnosis. This immediately raises a difficult point. Traditional medicine depends upon the logical assessment of signs and symptoms produced by the patient in order that a label or diagnosis can be applied. A treatment is then selected which, from experience, we know tends to help people with that label. Unfortunately, this process can fail because the signs and symptoms may falsely suggest another label and so lead to a wrong treatment, as the patient may present with a confusing or 'non-labellable' condition.

It seems logical to many practitioners of alternative medicine (and aromatherapists are no exception) to cut out the middle or labelling phase and go straight to the treatment phase. In aromatherapy, many practitioners use radiesthesia to ascertain the best treatment for the patient. A pendulum is used to decide which remedy (in the form of essential oils) is appropriate for the patient and then the oil or combination of oils is prepared and administered. An actual diagnosis does not necessarily have to be made, provided the treatment matches the patient's needs exactly.

As we have seen, there are several ways of getting the

Some common ailments and their suggested aromatherapy remedies

Acne Bergamot, cajuput, camphor, cedarwood, juniper, lavender, sandalwood

Aphrodisiacs Black pepper, cardamom, clary sage, jasmine, juniper, orange blossom, patchouli, rose, sandalwood, ylang-ylang

Asthma Benzoin, cajuput, cypress, eucalyptus, hyssop, lavender, lemon, marjoram, melissa, origanum, pennyroyal, peppermint, pine, rosemary, sage, thyme

Bronchitis Basil, benzoin, bergamot, cajuput, camphor, cardamom, cedarwood, eucalyptus, frankincense, hyssop, lavender, pennyroyal, peppermint, pine, rosemary, sandalwood, terebinth, thyme

Burns Camphor, chamomile, eucalyptus, geranium, lavender, rosemary, sage

Colds Basil, black pepper, camphor, eucalyptus, marjoram, melissa, pennyroyal, peppermint, rosemary

Colic Benzoin, bergamot, black pepper, camphor, cardamom, chamomile, clary sage, fennel, hyssop, juniper, lavender, marjoram, melissa, peppermint

Constipation Black pepper, camphor, fennel, marjoram, rose, rosemary, terebinth

Cough Benzoin, black pepper, cardamom, cypress, eucalyptus, frankincense, hyssop, jasmine, juniper, myrrh, pennyroyal, peppermint, sandalwood

Cystitis Benzoin, cajuput, cedarwood, eucalyptus, fennel, juniper, lavender, pine, sandalwood, terebinth, thyme

Depression Basil, bergamot, camphor, chamomile, clary sage, geranium, jasmine, lavender, melissa, orange blossom, patchouli, rose, sandalwood, ylang-ylang

Diarrhoea Black pepper, camphor, chamomile, cinnamon, clove, cypress, eucalyptus, geranium, juniper, lavender, lemon, myrrh, orange, orange blossom, peppermint, rosemary, sage, sandalwood

Eczema Bergamot, chamomile, geranium, hyssop, juniper, lavender, sage

Fainting Basil, black pepper, chamomile, lavender, melissa, pennyroyal, peppermint, rosemary, sage, thyme

Fever Basil, bergamot, black pepper, camphor, chamomile, eucalyptus, hyssop, lemon, melissa, pennyroyal

Flatulence Bergamot, black pepper, camphor, cardamom, chamomile, cinnamon, clary sage, clove, coriander, fennel, hyssop, juniper, lavender, lemon, marjoram, myrrh, pennyroyal, peppermint, rosemary, sage, terebinth, thyme

Haemorrhoids Cypress, frankincense, juniper, melissa

Headaches cardamon, chamomile, lavender, lemon, marjoram, pennyroyal, peppermint, rose, rosemary

Indigestion Basil, bergamot, black pepper, cardamom, chamomile, cinnamon, clary sage, clove, coriander, eucalyptus, fennel, frankincense, hyssop, juniper, lavender, lemon, lemongrass, marjoram, melissa, myrrh, pennyroyal, peppermint, rosemary, sage, thyme

Influenza Black pepper, cinnamon, cypress, eucalyptus, hyssop, lavender, lemon, peppermint, pine, rosemary, sage, thyme

Mental fatigue Basil, cardamom, clove, peppermint, rosemary, thyme

Mouth ulcers Myrrh, pennyroyal

Nausea Basil, black pepper, cardamom, fennel, lavender, lemon, melissa, peppermint, rose, sandalwood

Nervous tension Benzoin, bergamot, camphor, chamomile, cypress, geranium, jasmine, lavender, marjoram, melissa, orange blossom, patchouli, rose, sandalwood, ylang-ylang

Rheumatism Cajuput, camphor, chamomile, eucalyptus, hyssop, juniper, lavender,

origanum, pine, rosemary, terebinth, thyme

Sedatives Benzoin, bergamot, camphor, cedarwood, chamomile, clary sage, cypress, frankincense, geranium, hyssop, jasmine, juniper, lavender, marjoram, melissa, myrrh, orange blossom, patchouli, rose, sandalwood, ylang-ylang

Shock Camphor, melissa, orange blossom, peppermint

Sinusitis Cajuput, eucalyptus, peppermint, pine

Skin – dry Chamomile, geranium, jasmine, lavender, orange blossom, rose, sandalwood, ylang-ylang

Skin – oily Bergamot, camphor, cedarwood, cypress, frankincense, geranium, juniper, lavender, lemon, orange, sandalwood, ylang-ylang

Skin – mature Benzoin, clary sage, cypress, frankincense, lavender, myrrh, orange blossom, patchouli, rose

Skin – sensitive Chamomile, jasmine, orange blossom, rose

Sore throat Clary sage, eucalyptus, geranium, lavender, sage

Stimulants Black pepper, camphor, eucalyptus, pennyroyal, peppermint, rosemary

Toothache Cajuput, camphor, chamomile, clove, pennyroyal, peppermint, sage

beneficial effects of aromatic oils. Some aromatherapists use the essences orally as if they were traditional medicines, some use inhalations and others apply the oil to the skin. Some therapists use a combination of all three.

If the oils are to be absorbed via the skin, there are other factors that come into play. First, the skin has to be cleaned and receptive to the oils. Many people's skins are not receptive simply because modern diets, make-up and environmental pollutants have reduced the skin from being a vital organ to a semi-inert covering of the body. A good aromatherapist will spend much time cleaning and preparing the skin for therapy and will encourage the oils to penetrate by very hot compresses, aromatic baths, warming lamps, Swedish massage, 'osteopathic' massage or even acupuncture.

By using one or more of these methods the oils are encouraged to pass through the skin, so treating the local condition, stimulating or relaxing the patient and at the same time having effects elsewhere in the body by treating meridians or reflex zones (see page 288). It has been found from experience that massaging the face or back is usually sufficient to achieve the desired results. A series of about ten treatments is usually necessary although results can be seen more quickly.

What is it used for?

Many conditions are said to improve with the use of essential oils but the most dramatic improvements are said to be seen in wound healing, scar resorption, acne, stretch marks from pregnancy (which can be prevented with the right oils) and many stress-orientated states. The treatments are at best a clever herbal cure with very little danger from side-effects or toxicity and at worst a pleasantly relaxing massage combined with simple supportive psychotherapy from the aromatherapist.

Aromatherapy will never be very popular simply because of the cost. Essential oils are extremely expensive to buy and have to be stored in critical conditions to ensure they retain their potency. The matching of therapy to patient is a skill that takes years to perfect and a long time to work out for each individual patient. As the therapy is time-consuming and uses expensive raw materials it is unlikely to become a popular alternative medicine for the masses.

Does it work?

Undoubtedly the answer is 'yes', if practised by an experienced therapist and for the rather limited range of conditions I've outlined above. It's difficult to be sure whether the aromatic oils themselves (which are after all what aromatherapy is all about) do as much as is claimed. Certainly they can and do penetrate the skin, especially with massage and heat but quite what they do then is not so easy to prove. They may well have effects on certain organs, but a lot more research needs to be done to be sure that the substances supposedly so useful in curative terms don't also have adverse effects.

Unfortunately such research will be a very long time coming because it is so expensive and difficult to do. There is only a handful of plant biochemists in Britain for example who have the kind of expertise to be able to work on such minute fractions of plant cells. The only way that the essential oils are likely to be studied in greater depth is if the pharmaceutical industry with its massive research budgets decides to put real effort into such research. In the present climate this is unlikely to happen but may come about as medicines become harder and more expensive to discover and as the public demands more 'natural' forms of therapy.

Ayurveda

Definition

Arguably the most ancient of all medical disciplines. A system of sacred medicine dating back to Ancient India from which most western medicine is derived.

Background

Oriental therapy, of which Ayurveda is a part, is very ancient – dating from 1000 to 3000 BC. It probably all started in the Nile and Euphrates valleys. It is widely held that much of our western medicine originated in ancient Greece. This is true as far as it goes but the Greeks learned much in turn from the Indians. Hindu medical classics are said to contain no technical terms that point to a foreign origin, whereas the ideas and many of the drugs used by the Greeks are of Middle Eastern and Indian origin. A leading expert who has spent years studying the subject has come to the conclusion that Pythagoras (who indirectly affected so much of the teaching of Hippocrates – who has been called the father of western medicine) took his whole system directly from India. So it looks very much as though most of our medical knowledge originated in India.

Ayurveda (ayur means 'life' and veda, 'knowledge' or 'science'), the science of life, is a later addition to an ancient Hindu sacred writing dating from 1200 BC – the Artharva-veda. The first known school to teach Ayurvedic medicine was at the University of Banaras in about 500 BC. It was here that the great *Samhita* or encyclopaedia of medicine was written. Seven hundred years later another great encyclopaedia was written and these two between them form the basis of Ayurveda.

This school of medicine is responsible for the health care of 80–90 per cent of the people of India today although there are extremely few practitioners in the West. But Ayurveda is worth looking at because it is almost certainly the most ancient school of medical thought still in practice today and because many of the other systems, including very ancient Chinese and Japanese disciplines, arose from it.

What is it?

It's very difficult to get a contemporary view of Ayurveda because the vast majority of Indian doctors who come to the West are so westernized that they have lost touch with the deeper meaning of Ayurveda. Also, over three thousand years, the very nature of Ayurveda has changed as Man has increasingly demanded physical explanations for things and wanted to reduce everything to the laws of physics and chemistry. Indian metaphysics and yoga are now enjoying a considerable following in the West so perhaps we are slowly becoming more able to accept or at least be more open to other medical philosophies.

According to Ayurvedic medicine, at the level of the individual mind there are three types of activity, Rajas, Tamas and Satva, which correspond to active creating energy, passive destroying or resisting energy and unifying, preserving energy. Similarly it describes Pitta, the active energy of heat, Kapha, the element of phlegm (which is cold) and Vayu, the element air.

These three energies are modified by three processes – spiritual, mental and physical. The human being and the universe are composed of five elements called Bhutas. *Ether* is all around and equivalent to sound; *air* is light and equivalent to touch; *fire* is hot, gives colour and is equivalent to sight; *water* is flowing, wet and equivalent to taste; *earth* is heavy, moist and equivalent to smell. This is on a parallel with the four formative forces of Rudolf Steiner (see page 93) and the Four Humours of the ancient Greeks. Ether or air is regarded as common to all these systems.

According to Ayurveda, the human body is made up of seven tissues – the Dhatus – and so long as these are in balance, the person is healthy. Food, once digested, feeds the seven Dhatus but any imbalance in the food produces disease in them. Although Ayurveda puts great emphasis on wrong food as a cause of disease, it also acknowledges that physical activity, sleep, sexual habits, the climate, emotional states, physical surroundings, age and sex all influence disease.

How is it done?

Ayurveda doesn't rely on making a diagnosis as we understand it in the West. The Ayurvedic doctor tries to treat the patient as a whole, because the basis of the system is that each person is a unique individual and subject to unique imbalances in his life. The history-taking phase of the medical assessment includes astrological considerations and in addition to a thorough physical examination the physician will examine urine, sweat, sputum and the patient's voice.

Unlike other medical systems, Ayurveda expects the patient to play his part in his cure. 'Recollection, obedience to instructions, courage and ability to describe his ailments are considered necessary in a patient', according to one of the great encyclopaedias. Fasting, baths, applications to the skin, cleansing diets, enemas and blood-letting are all used to cleanse the body before superimposing any specific treatment. Drugs are given to bring all the Dhatus and other bodily systems into balance again. The pharmacopoeia of drugs is very refined and enormous in size which is scarcely surprising after so many thousands of years of development. Ayurveda also includes the use of mantras (repeated prayer-like utterings), ceremonies, yogic breathing and other techniques. All the drugs are prepared by the individual practitioner and given as jellies, tinctures, powders, pills or oils. Refined metallic and mineral oxides and oxides of precious stones are also held in high esteem.

Ayurveda doesn't only have a place in the management of internal disease though – there are branches of surgery, obstetrics, gynaecology, paediatrics and psychology just as in the West. Ayurveda also deals especially thoroughly with sexual disorders.

It's important to bear in mind that Ayurveda is not a physical system of medicine like that of the West. Its origins are sacred and it operates at all levels in Man. Other fringe medicines such as homoeopathy (see page 175), colour therapy (see page 141) and radiesthesia (see page 261) are linked to and possibly derived from Ayurveda. It is a way of life but far too metaphysical for most westerners even to begin to grasp. Like so many of the more erudite and elegant systems of medicine of the past, Ayurveda demands much of its practitioners too. Today's concept of a doctor who does a 'job' of healing people and then goes off to play golf would be hard to accept for the Ayurvedic practitioner, to whom his science, religious beliefs and medical practice are a total way of life.

Bach Remedies

Definition

A system of herbal medical remedies devised by Edward Bach (1880–1936).

Background

Edward Bach was a medical practitioner who worked in London at University College Hospital as a bacteriologist. The hospital announced that its staff had to work full time there or not at all, so Bach left to become Pathologist and Bacteriologist to the London Homoeopathic Hospital. In 1926 he wrote a book, *Chronic Disease: A Working Hypothesis*, in collaboration with Dr C. E. Wheeler and soon grew so busy that he left the hospital to run his own laboratories and large Harley Street practice.

Suddenly he threw up his lucrative practice and retired to Wales to search for flowers and trees that had healing powers. In the last years of his life he discovered thirty-eight herbal remedies which he developed from herbs found in England, Wales and continental Europe. In 1931 he published *Heal Thyself – an explanation of the real causes and cure of disease. The Twelve Healers* appeared in 1933. He fell into disfavour with the General Medical Council because he advertised his cures, but was not struck off the medical register.

As with most pioneers, his life was not made easy. His medical colleagues thought he had 'gone off his head' and his friends despaired at the loss of a man of real talent to the medical profession. Dr Bach knew he was doing the right thing and continued testing his remedies on himself. He was a frail man and died in 1936 at the age of fifty-six.

What are Bach remedies?

Bach proved, at least to his own satisfaction, that warmed dew absorbed the properties of the plant from whose surface it was collected. As the collection of dew was so tedious when it came to producing these remedies in any quantity, he tried putting flowers in a glass bowl of pure spring water and leaving it to stand in the full sun for a few hours. He found that this was a very effective way of impregnating the water with the power of the plant. He then bottled the water with some brandy for preservation purposes. Out of this stock bottle he took a few drops and added them to one ounce bottles of pure water. The patient then took four drops of this diluted remedy in a little water four times a day. If the remedy called for buds, stalks or certain leaves, the plant material was boiled in water for half an hour and then stock solutions prepared as before.

These floral remedies, he claimed, could alter the disharmonies of personality and emotional state that trouble us all from time to time. In other words his remedies were mostly aimed at curing emotional states rather than physical ones. For example, if you suffered from fearfulness, you took mimulus; indecision was treated with scleranthus; lack of faith with gentian; and obsessional thoughts with white chestnut. He also used his remedies to relieve ordinary physical conditions and devised a combination of five of the remedies as a cure-all for any emergency situation. This he called the Rescue Remedy.

How is it done?

There are only a few practitioners anywhere following the remarkable work of Edward Bach but those who use his remedies speak very highly of them. Dr Alec Forbes, a very experienced physician in Plymouth, England, uses them regularly. He uses remedies that he knows from experience work in particular emotional states, but started by using the remedies for the indications given by Dr Bach and other practitioners who have written on the subject. His experience of the remedies over many years is that they are as effective at ridding patients of their emotional problems as any of the pharmaceutical products he uses and have the advantage of extremely low cost and almost no problems. Bach used his remedies mostly for patients with depression, anxiety or schizophrenia and Forbes has good results with these very same categories of patients. He advises the patient slowly to withdraw the drugs he's taking as the Bach remedy takes effect. 'Most of these people are only too anxious to get off the drugs,' he claims, 'because they don't like their side-effects and are afraid of taking them in the long term.' Forbes finds that about 70 per cent of such patients get better with Bach remedies and at one tenth the cost of drugs. Very occasionally Bach remedies produce symptoms but these usually result from premature or sudden stopping of the drugs that the patient was previously taking. They are really withdrawal symptoms. Physical side-effects don't occur with the Bach remedies. There is no accurate dose of the remedies – the therapist is guided by results and varies the dose accordingly.

Another English doctor who uses Bach remedies found he had to use another way of deciding which remedy to use in which patient. 'I took the patient's left hand in my right, then, after a short interval to get "attuned", working blindly, I took up each remedy in turn with my left hand, running through the whole thirty-eight. On some I got a reaction, i.e. a sort of tingling sensation which started at the back of my scalp and, if strong, would go all over me. If I got this reaction on a bottle, I put it aside. At the end I looked to see which bottles I had put aside and took it that these were what the patient needed. The numbers chosen varied from one to six, seldom more.' He found that this method of divining the treatment the patient needed was surprisingly accurate as judged by the subsequent cures. On occasions this procedure led him to make a diagnosis and gain insight into the patient which he would otherwise never have gained without the Bach remedy diagnosis.

Why do they work?

In short, nobody knows but we can be sure it is nothing to do with any chemicals that leak out of the flower into the water. Analysis of the water shows that there is no perceivable difference between the water before and after the flower has been left in it in the sunshine. The answer seems to lie in the transfer of some of the 'forces' of the plant itself – the 'flower power' – into the water molecules. In a sense this is akin to homoeopathic theory but without the succussion or trituration that is used in homoeopathy. Dr Forbes asserts that the plant material transfers its unique pattern to the water in some as yet inexplicable way. He tells of a doctor he knows who can work exactly similar cures as those obtained with Bach remedies by giving the patient a piece of paper with the name of the remedy written on it or by writing the name of the remedy on the patient's skin with a blunt instrument.

Clearly there's an enormous amount of research yet to be done into Bach remedies but unfortunately it is very difficult to do in the classical double blind trial so beloved of the medical profession.

Could it all be a sort of clever psychotherapy?

'That's very unlikely', says Dr Forbes, 'because I don't go out of my way to do anything psychotherapeutically with either group of patients (those who are on drugs or those on the remedies) yet the results from the remedies are every bit as good as those I get with drugs.'

Biochemics

Definition

A system of medical therapy devised in the last century by a German doctor and chemist, Dr Wilhelm Heinrich Schuessler, based on the premise that every form of illness is associated with disturbances of the balance of one or several of the body's inorganic salts.

Background

Dr Schuessler, a doctor in the middle of the last century, became disenchanted with what he could offer his patients and so turned to homoeopathy. He was influenced in his thinking by the great chemist Liebig, by Hahnemann, the father of homoeopathy, and by Virchow who showed that the body consisted of individual cells composed of organic materials, water and inorganic salts. Experiments at the time showed that twelve basic chemical salts were common to all cremated bodies and Schuessler spent years proving by experimentation that these twelve salts were essential to maintain health.

He set about discovering which salts were needed for each disease process and in so doing gave birth to a branch of fringe medicine now called biochemics. Companies all over the world now make his twelve biochemic tissue salts for sale to doctors and the public alike. Under the influence of Hahnemann, Schuessler gave the tissue salts in homoeopathic doses and he found they were useful clinical tools. Since Schuessler's time, a well-known English biochemics expert, Dr Eric Powell, has claimed that there are a further thirty salts essential as trace elements in the body and other workers in the field have found and used yet others.

Biochemic salts are used in the USA and the UK and very widely in Asia (particularly India), Germany and France and they are available at the homoeopathic pharmacies that abound in France.

What are these salts?

Dr Schuessler's Biochemic System of Medicine revolves around the following inorganic salts: calcium fluoride (Calc. Fluor.); calcium phosphate (Calc. Phos.); calcium sulphate (Calc. Sulph.); iron phosphate (Ferr. Phos.); potassium chloride (Kali. Mur.); potassium phosphate (Kali. Phos.); potassium sulphate (Kali. Sulph.); magnesium phosphate (Mag. Phos.); sodium chloride (Nat. Mur.); sodium phosphate (Nat. Phos.); sodium sulphate (Nat. Sulph.); and silicon oxide (Silica). The table shows some commonly used combinations and the indications for their use:

A **Ferr. Phos., Kali. Phos., Mag. Phos.** Neuralgia, neuritis, sciatica and allied conditions

B **Calc. Phos., Kali. Phos., Ferr. Phos.** General debility, nervous exhaustion and during convalescence

C **Mag. Phos., Nat. Phos., Nat. Sulph., Silica** Acidity, dyspepsia, heartburn and allied conditions

D **Kali. Mur., Kali. Sulph., Calc. Sulph., Silica** Minor skin ailments and allied conditions

E **Calc. Phos., Mag. Phos., Nat. Phos., Nat. Sulph.** Flatulence, colic, indigestion and allied conditions

F **Kali. Phos., Mag. Phos., Nat. Mur., Silica** Migraine, nervous headache and allied conditions

G **Calc. Fluor., Calc. Phos., Kali. Phos., Nat. Mur.** Backache, lumbago, piles and allied conditions

H **Mag. Phos., Nat. Mur., Silica** Hay fever and allied conditions

I **Ferr. Phos., Kali. Sulph., Mag. Phos.** Fibrositis, muscular pain and allied conditions

How is it done?

Biochemics is based on the principle that all symptoms and signs are caused by a lack of one of twelve inorganic salts. Biochemics is essentially a form of self-help, so the first thing the patient has to do is to be sure of the symptoms and signs he has. Biochemics experts claim that a lack of any one salt usually corresponds fairly accurately with a group of symptoms. In order to treat the symptoms, the patient takes that particular salt. Iron phosphate deficiency is associated with inflammation; spasmodic pains and cramps with magnesium phosphate deficiency; acidity with sodium phosphate and so on. As a disease changes so the remedies should be changed to cope with each new symptom, it is claimed. Some people suffer from the cumulative effects of long term drug administration or other abuse of their bodies and in such cases the response to biochemic remedies may be slow.

Some conditions need several salts to produce the desired result. These are usually taken singly at thirty minute intervals. The frequency and regularity of dosage is all important. The tablets should be taken every half hour if the case is acute and, in less urgent cases, every two hours during the day. Some of the remedies can be applied externally, for example sodium chloride for insect bites. Biochemic salts are claimed by their followers to be excellent first aid standbys.

How do they work?

Schuessler's tissue salts work in much the same way that any homoeopathic remedy works (see page 175) because they are all produced homoeopathically. In fact biochemics is really a branch of homoeopathy. It is, however, a branch that doesn't please some homoeopaths because they believe that remedies should aim at normalizing imbalances in the body and shouldn't be taken simply as 'symptom relievers' or as a first aid measure. It seems to me that for common self-limiting ailments biochemics may well work to the benefit of the patient but, as with any kind of self-medication, it's essential that the patient reports to a doctor any sign or symptom that seems to persist for more than a few days in spite of biochemic treatment.

Apparently people who take biochemic salts (and there are lots of them – one UK company alone sells millions of bottles a year) learn which salt or combination of salts works best for them under certain conditions. They thus develop their own first aid kit of tissue salts and stick to them, only going to doctors when the salts don't work. As with other self-prescribing that goes on all the time it is quite acceptable provided serious conditions aren't overlooked. Hopefully though self-medication with tissue salts will be less harmful than that which takes place with other products currently available over the pharmacist's counter. As they are homoeopathic remedies they probably in fact treat the underlying imbalances that are producing the patient's symptoms and so are perhaps not so reprehensible as many homoeopaths claim but it seems to me that it must take some skill, intelligence and patience to work out which salt is best for any given condition.

> THOSE WHO PRACTISE BIOCHEMICS
> HAVE FAITH IN THE SALTS AND
> CLAIM
> CONSIDERABLE RESULTS WITH THEM

There is no experimental evidence comparable with normal clinical trials on drugs that these salts work but anecdotal evidence abounds and it's tempting to believe that the millions of people who buy them actually use them and find them of value.

Those who practise biochemics (and most of them are homoeopaths – both medically and non-medically trained) have faith in the salts and claim considerable results with them. Until much more study is carried out it is impossible to say how they work but in many cases they undoubtedly do. But even those who use them with success will agree that there sometimes comes a point

Biochemic remedies available at health food stores and chemists

Combination A for neuritis, sciatica
Combination B for edginess, exhaustion, convalescence
Combination C for acidity, heartburn, dyspepsia
Combination D for minor skin ailments
Combination E for flatulence, indigestion, colic
Combination F for nervous and migraine headache
Combination G for backache, lumbago
Combination H for hayfever
Combination I for fibrositis, muscular pain
Combination J for coughs, colds, chestiness
Combination K for brittle nails
Combination L for oxygenation of tissues
Combination M for rheumatic conditions
Combination N for menstrual pain
Combination P for aching feet and legs, chilblains
Combination Q for catarrh, sinus disorders
Combination R for infants' teething pains
Combination S for biliousness, stomach upsets

when pharmaceutical preparations are essential. Tissue salts have their shortcomings – like all medicines – but as a self-help, first aid kit, they are probably as good as anything available and a lot safer than most.

Biofeedback

Definition

A method by which the body's functions can be monitored using equipment specially designed for the purpose in order to enable a person to gain control over himself by giving him information he would not otherwise be able to obtain.

Background

The term 'feedback' originates from the radio industry at the beginning of the century when it was defined by Norbert Wiener, a founder of research into feedback, as 'a method of controlling a system by reinserting into it the results of its past performance'. We are all feeding back information into our nervous systems every moment of our lives whether we realize it or not. All our biological systems feed information to the brain which subsequently modifies the next reaction or action in the light of these experiences.

Biofeedback as used in medicine is a young discipline, probably only some twenty years old, that grew out of operant condition training in animals. The subject started off in the hands of psychologists but soon became of interest to the medical profession which reasoned that some of the lessons learned from animal work could usefully be applied to Man. At first the signals being fed back were relatively unsophisticated but the work of Joe Kamiya in the USA took the subject a whole stage further with his almost accidental discovery in 1958 that man could control his own brain activity. He found that he could train people to produce a special sort of brain wave (alpha rhythm). He devised a piece of electrical apparatus that transformed brain waves into an auditory signal so that each time the subject produced alpha waves he would hear a tone. The subject's task thereafter was to sustain the tone. Most people trained in this way can learn to produce alpha brain waves within a few hours. The interesting thing is that most people associated alpha activity with a sense of pleasure and well-being which thus opened up possibilities for making people feel less anxious and more relaxed. Biofeedback of brain waves also means that we can now measure the EEG changes associated with mental states such as hate, envy, depression, ecstasy and so on. Today it's not only alpha waves that can be measured and influenced – many other brain waves can be too. Alpha waves are associated with feelings of relaxation and well-being as we have seen. Beta waves are dominant when the person is aroused; theta with the appearance of spontaneous visual images; and delta waves with deep sleep or meditation states.

Biofeedback as a science is more properly called biofeedback *training* because it involves the positive training of the body to modify specific activities with the benefit of experience. The very thought of being able actively to control one's heart beat, for instance, or the rate at which blood flows through a kidney is so alien to us in the West that many of us are tempted to reject biofeedback before knowing anything more of it. As westerners, we are not taught to look inwards, to visualize our internal organs. On the contrary we are brought up with a feeling of distaste and disgust for what goes on inside us. The yogi at the other extreme visualizes all his organs and bodily functions (which are as real to him as his fingers) and controls them at will. This seems like magic at first but can be explained along modern neurophysiological lines, as we shall see.

Until less than ten years ago it was generally believed that Man was controlled by two distinct nervous systems. One was the voluntary system (the one that makes all deliberate and controlled movement possible) and the other the involuntary one (which controlled the vital 'background ' bodily functions like the heartbeat, breathing, blood flow and so on). Professor Neal E. Miller of New York's Rockefeller University set out against fearful odds to prove that this distinction was a false one in the late 1960s. Working on rats paralysed with curare he was able to teach them to control their automatic responses and to do so very accurately. One rat for example could increase the blood flow to each ear on demand. This work has now been extended to man and experiments using electroencephalograms and electrocardiograms have shown that people can be trained to control minute fractions of brain or heart activity.

But what biofeedback has done above almost anything is to revive in the simplistic and sceptical West a sense of respect for the power of the human mind. At last we can prove that man is capable of 'willing' things to happen. Biofeedback experts the world over can, for example, train a person to increase a particular type of brain wave (alpha waves) that occurs in us all, in such a way as to make the subject feel relaxed and pleasant. This opens up a whole new horizon in mind training and possibly heralds the dawning of an era less reliant on drugs.

Once we get into this field more deeply we can begin to understand how many previously inexplicable phenomena work. Take placebo activity, for example. If a doctor gives a patient an inactive tablet and tells him it's a drug, a certain percentage of people will experience what they are told to expect. Patients given a sickness-inducing drug in one survey, after they had been told that it would cure their vomiting, did in fact stop vomiting. Approximately 35 per cent of the physically ill and 40 per cent of the mentally ill respond to placebos, a fact which is often used in the practice of modern medicine. It's interesting to note that in a recent survey in which patients with pain were treated with placebos, it was found that red placebos were most effective of all and were even more effective than a real pain-killer that had been included in the trial!

A knowledge of biofeedback might also explain why it is that people die very soon after the death of a spouse and how others can will themselves to live or die under exactly similar clinical situations. Any physician can recount a host of stories to illustrate the power the mind has over the body in this way but it wasn't until recently that this was able to be proved. Sociologist David Phillips made some interesting discoveries about Yom Kippur, the Jewish Day of Atonement, and those who observe it. He found that there was a notable drop in death rate just before this important day in the Jewish calendar and that there was no similar drop for non-Jews in this period. He also found a drop in death rate before birthdays and a significant peak of deaths afterwards – all of which seem to show that 'Some people look forward to witnessing certain important occasions and are able to put off dying in order to do so.'

Biofeedback is the subject of hundreds of papers in medical and psychological literature and is gaining enormous popularity in the United States although it is still somewhat embryonic there. Things are not much more advanced anywhere although there are a few practitioners in the UK and the Netherlands and isolated centres of interest elsewhere.

As with so many advances in medicine, biofeedback caught on because it was in the right place at the right time. The discovery that Man could by his own will alter the functioning of his internal organs came at a time when there was a tremendous interest in meditation, yoga and other similar pursuits. With the Beatles interesting themselves in the world of the supernatural in the full public gaze and with the ripples on the US pond spreading from the pebbles dropped in California, it wasn't long before even quite ordinary middle-class people were talking about and doing things they would have considered freaky only a few years before. There has been an enormous growth in the self-awareness movement and biofeedback was there to record it. In a strange way biofeedback combines the virtues of meditation with those of the latest in electronic gadgetry. As such it must have a sound future.

How is it done?

Basically biofeedback training is simple in concept. The doctor uses some kind of electrical or electronic instrument to monitor a particular output from a patient and then displays it in such a way as to allow the patient to appreciate changes in the output.

At the simplest level, a fingertip blood flow meter or perspiration meter might be used. The patient is wired up and then subjected to stimuli so as to help him achieve the desired effect. If, for example, the equipment is wired up in such a way as to record greater relaxation, blood flow, or whatever is being measured as a number of lights on a board, then the patient will be asked to do something to try to make the lights go out. The doctor will either talk reassuringly to the patient (one doctor I know reads beautiful passages of relaxing prose to her patients), ask him to concentrate on or 'visualize' helpful scenes, or even frankly reward the patient when he gets things right. Anything goes so long as it achieves the desired effect.

The following is a good example of a reward-orientated biofeedback system. Dr David Shapiro of Harvard Medical School has used biofeedback training to help patients control their high blood pressure. The subject is seated in a cubicle with pre-set levels of light and sound and a blood pressure cuff is wrapped around his arm. Once the test has started, the patient's instructions are to keep the red light shining, together with an accompanying sound. He is told that the machine is wired up in such a way that the more frequently the red light flashes on, the better he is controlling his blood pressure. Every time he builds up a score of twenty flashes of the red light, he's 'rewarded' with a five second flash of a *Playboy* nude pin-up. Subjects rapidly learned how to control their blood pressure using this method.

But this delightful piece of research highlights a potential problem with biofeedback in general – the possibility that the subject will only respond to the situation as produced in the laboratory. Because of this, some doctors in the field use a minimum of gadgetry but encourage the patient to visualize things that make the biofeedback equipment respond as desired. By interiorizing the feedback stimulus in this way, they maintain it is easier to get people to do these desired routines in the kitchen at home or in the car on the way to work.

Of course the ideal would be to be able to have one's own biofeedback machine which one could use at home so that one could keep on practising without the help of a doctor or trainer. Such equipment is available fairly inexpensively. There are four main types that can be bought. The first of these is an EEG machine (electroencephalograph) which records alpha waves from the brain. Caution has to be used with this type of equipment because blinking, tensing the muscles of the forehead, twitching, frowning or gritting the teeth can all cause apparently increased alpha rhythms. Thus an inexperienced person using this equipment at home would be misinterpreting the alpha wave activity and so be perpetuating bad old habits rather than creating good new ones.

EMG equipment (a myophone that measures muscle tension is one type) appears to be better than an EEG machine for domestic use but it's important that the underlying physical malfunction has been properly diagnosed first. For example, a 'tension headache' could be a brain tumour and no good at all would be done by wiring up to the biofeedback machine if this is the case. Such machines should only ever be used *after* a consultation with a doctor to rule out serious, treatable disease. With this proviso, the EMG, which registers muscular activity, can be a very useful tool.

The Relaxometer, a straightforward galvanic resistance machine, is attached to the fingertips and is simple to use. It is also very safe and cheap. This instrument measures skin-resistance (which varies according to the amount of sweat on the fingertip under the electrode) and provides feedback via an auditory signal which varies from a low buzz to a high whine. The more tense the subject, the higher the whine. The Relaxometer is not to be confused with the E meter – long used by scientologists. Certainly they work on the same principle but with the E meter only the observer knows the response of the subject – there is thus no feedback.

Lastly, temperature feedback equipment. Here again, this should be used only after consultation with a doctor. 'Temperature trainers' register blood flow in the underlying tissues and show promise in the treatment of cases of Raynaud's disease and migraine.

But all this equipment, be it in a laboratory or in the home, is only a way of training the person to control his bodily functions at will. The idea is to become so trained that eventually no machines are required and the desired effects are obtained on a daily basis as a normal part of the person's life.

What is it used for?

Many claims have been made for biofeedback training and many are bogus or frankly short term money makers. Medically though there is now an enormous body of evidence (almost entirely from the USA) that supports the use of biofeedback actually to cure and prevent disease.

Using biofeedback training the patient and doctor together find a way for the patient to help himself back to health. Many of our contemporary ailments are linked to stress or rather the bottling up of repressed emotions which, in a more primitive society, would have found an outlet in aggression of some kind. Stress-orientated diseases do well with biofeedback. Anxiety is therefore one of the areas that was first looked at and indeed is a condition in which good results can be claimed. The idea here is simply to get the patient to relax. Most people find this very difficult and need to be taught how to do it. Respiration biofeedback, in which a patient listens to his own amplified breath sounds, is a new method that seems to be more helpful than simple instructions to relax. Other doctors in the USA have attached electrodes to muscles and fed the impulses back to an EMG machine. But however the relaxation is induced or recorded, the end result is much the same – a measurable fall in anxiety levels as gauged by objective testing.

In the USA, migraine and tension headaches, high blood pressure, insomnia, muscular tics, heart disease and psychiatric diseases have all been treated using biofeedback training. Doctors in Britain have used it to help with relaxation training for childbirth; in the treatment of addiction to smoking, eating and drinking; to cure stammering; and to help with migraine (one clinic in Birmingham found that 80 per cent of sufferers were improved).

As a science it is still in its infancy. Biofeedback is opening doors to the power of the mind over physical disease. Some doctors are looking at the possibility of using biofeedback to diagnose brain disorders in the USA and others see a possible future in being able to reverse certain neuroses using this method. Hyperactive children are being trained to control their alpha brain waves in a school for problem children in Texas, with the result that they are calmer and have fewer problems with insomnia and stuttering without the use of tranquillizers. In several laboratories in the USA, epileptic patients are being trained to suppress certain abnormal brain waves but this is still a long way off actually preventing epileptic fits.

Whether it is via brain waves, muscle tension, or some other type of biofeedback, here is a science with a great deal to offer in the future. Some workers look to the day when a patient with an ulcer will be taught how to control the production of acid by his stomach. Others have even suggested that 'voluntary starvation and absorption of cancerous growths through blood flow control might be found to be feasible'. Another way that cancers could possibly be helped by biofeedback training is by reducing the person's stress level. Fear produces a stress reaction which causes increased amounts of stress hormones to be produced and this in turn switches off the body's natural immunity to some extent. By alleviating fear and stress, biofeedback training might thus be able to help the body's own defences cope better with a growth.

Voluntary control of blood flow, such as can be achieved with biofeedback, already looks like being useful in the treatment of Raynaud's disease, a condition in which the hands have a poor circulation.

The future holds a lot of exciting possibilities for biofeedback – we have only just opened the door.

Chiropractic

Definition

An entirely manipulative therapy designed to maintain the spinal column and nervous system in good health without the use of surgery or drugs.

Background

The word chiropractic comes from the Greek words *cheir* – hands, and *praktikos* – done by, thus chiropractic means 'done by the hand'.

Chiropractic is very old indeed. Ancient Egyptian manuscripts have descriptions of chiropractic techniques and the ancient Hindus, Chinese, Babylonians and Assyrians also used manipulative treatment. It fell into disuse and it wasn't until 1895 that it made its reappearance.

Today's understanding of chiropractic is based on the work of a Canadian, Dr Daniel David Palmer. His first success was with his janitor, Harvey Lilliard, whose deafness he cured by manipulating the vertebrae in his neck. Encouraged by this and other successes that followed, Palmer studied even more deeply the anatomical and physiological basis for such cures and soon evolved a philosophy and treatment which we call chiropractic. He carried out numerous experiments, recorded the results and began to create a real science of a previously woolly art.

Before long, Palmer had given up his old therapies (mainly mesmerism and magnetic healing) and devoted himself entirely to chiropractic. The word chiropractic was coined by one of Palmer's patients, a clergyman. Palmer founded and became first

President of the Palmer Infirmary and Chiropractic Institute in Iowa in the USA.

Since Palmer's day, chiropractic has had a chequered history. In almost every country (with the possible exception of Germany) it has in the past been poorly regarded by the orthodox medical profession and in the USA chiropractors were threatened with prison before chiropractic registration was introduced. Much of this opposition has been ill-informed because most doctors don't realize or accept that some health problems can be caused by interference with nerve transmission caused by slight deviations, called subluxations, of bony parts especially in the vertebral column.

In spite of opposition in most western countries, chiropractic continues to flourish but not nearly as well as it should, especially in the light of truly remarkable findings in a large study of chiropractic in Germany.

Chiropractors undergo a four year full-time training. They study many of the subjects that doctors do but obviously spend much more time learning about the spine.

The profession has spread rapidly since the days of Palmer and today there are more than 25,000–30,000 chiropractors in the USA and Canada alone, where they practise legally under State and Provincial Law. Chiropractic is recognized in several Australian states, New Zealand and Switzerland. Denmark and Norway are in the process of legislating on the matter. In fact chiropractic is the most widely recognized alternative medical profession worldwide.

What is it?

Chiropractic is a skill in which joints are manipulated by hand in order to rebalance the body's function. Most often, it is the spinal joints which are manipulated. Just like osteopaths, chiropractors work from the basic principle that modern life produces abnormalities in the joints and the muscles because of the trauma, accidents, postural imbalances and mental and physical stress we all endure.

So a chiropractor tries, by manipulation of joints together with good advice on diet, exercise and rest, to get the patient back to normal. Sometimes, a chiropractor will advise other treatments such as posture training, massage, heat, or yoga but the basic aim is to restore normal health and function by physically manipulating areas that are affecting the nervous system. Chiropractic doesn't claim to be a panacea but simply an additional aid to medicine.

How is it done?

After taking a history of the complaint, a chiropractor examines the patient in much the same way a doctor would but pays special attention to the nervous systems and the spine, posture, muscular imbalances and tenderness. He may or may not use other modern diagnostic aids but will probably take X-rays of the areas under consideration. Most practitioners have their own X-ray equipment.

The nature of the treatment depends upon the type of condition being treated but often repeated visits are necessary, especially to remedy longstanding problems. Basically the chiropractor tries to do three things:

1. To correct distortions of posture
2. To restore reasonable function to spinal and pelvic joints
3. To remove any irritation of nerves which might be causing pain or disturbed function.

There are, of course, dangers with chiropractic just as with osteopathy and for this reason the reader should only ever go to a qualified person for treatment. In the USA, where chiropractors are legally recognized, their malpractice insurance premiums are substantially lower than those of physicians and surgeons – so overall they must be very safe.

What is it used for?

Chiropractic is mainly called upon to treat low back pain, slipped discs, neck pain, shoulder and arm pain, headaches and other musculo-skeletal pains. However, because of the effect of chiropractic treatment on the nervous system the most unlikely conditions can be helped. Some cases of migraine and many cases of headache are relieved, as are some cases of asthma, indigestion, arthritis, giddiness, certain emotional conditions and manifestations of stress.

Apart from these conditions, people constantly ask chiropractors if they can do anything for arthritis. 'Arthritis' covers a complex mixture of medical conditions and as such no quick answer is possible. Severe osteoarthritis with destruction of the joints will probably not respond to chiropractic but even some of these cases get relief if the dysfunction of the joint can be improved to some extent. Much of the pain in arthritis doesn't come so much from the bone and tissue destruction as from the compensatory muscle spasms and functional imbalances that surround the affected joints. Many less serious cases of arthritis can be helped by chiropractic as millions of grateful patients know. No good chiropractor will claim to be able to cure complaints once they are advanced and severe tissue changes have taken place.

In summary, then, chiropractic is valuable in skilled hands for a limited range of conditions. These conditions, however, form one of the major groups of ailments that affect mankind. It is a shame that conventional medicine doesn't try to embrace many of the sound principles of chiropractic on a far wider basis than at present. (For more details of a related therapy, see Osteopathy, page 231.)

Colour Therapy

Definition

The use of colour (usually in the form of coloured light) to produce beneficial or healing effects.

Background

Colour therapy isn't a recent fad; it is a very ancient pursuit. It was originally used in ancient Greece and in the Healing Temples of Light and Colour at Heliopolis in ancient Egypt. It has also been held in high esteem for thousands of years by the Indians and Chinese.

Colour affects man in many proven ways. Investigations into colour preferences, the effect of colour on concentration, performance, sense of physical and mental well-being and so on have been well researched over many years and there is increasing evidence of the use of colour in the areas of mental health, hospital recovery rooms and the stimulation of mentally retarded children.

The most popular colour is blue (about one third of people like blue best according to several surveys), followed by red (which is only half as popular as blue). The most hated colour, according to a survey in 1970 by Granger, a psychologist at Durham University, was yellow. 'Play Orbit' at the Institute of Contemporary Arts in London in 1970 consisted of intellectual toys and games in three differently coloured rooms. One was black, one green and the other yellow. In the yellow room all the playthings were getting broken or stolen but there was no similar trouble in the other two rooms. No explanation could be found

	0	5	10	15	20	25	30	35
None								
Black								
Brown								
Blue								
Turquoise								
Green								
Yellow								
Orange								
Red								
Violet								
White								
Silver								
Gold								

*Results of questionnaires on preferred colours and shapes –
Preferred colour; (next page) Preferred shape*

other than the colour of the room. This finding has led a leading British colour therapist to wonder whether there might not be more crime committed under different types of street lighting at night. Only further research will resolve questions such as these.

But it's not simply colours that affect us; the form of an object also has surprising effects. There are deep-rooted psychological implications of shapes generally and once we start to link shape to colour the whole subject becomes yet more complex. In a study of 1,100 people in England, Theo Gimbel, one of the country's leading colour therapists, not only confirmed that most people preferred blue but linked colour and form with fascinating

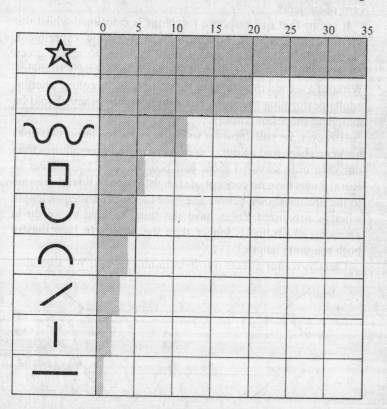

results. In his study he showed the subjects nine shapes, including simple straight lines, circles, curved lines and a pentagram.

The pentagram was favoured by more than a third of the group studied. This was followed by the circle (22·3 per cent) and the wave form (14·8 per cent). The simple lines were almost never chosen. When asked what colour they thought each shape should be, 38·8 per cent said the pentagram should be yellow. Only 2 per cent saw it as black. This is fascinating because the most popular shape by far was allotted the most unpopular colour by most of the respondents. Conversely, a horizontal line was seen as black by 37·6 per cent and as yellow by only 3·8 per cent of subjects.

It seems that our response to colour is emotional whilst our response to shape is intellectual. In a classic experiment, psychologist David Katz asked small children to match green discs against an assortment of red discs and green triangles. Without a second thought they matched them by colour whereas adults performing the same test asked whether they should be matching shapes or colours.

However, we still know far too little about the important links between shape and colour. Experiments with other cultures than our own only serve to show just how complex the subject is. Rural Zulus have no concept of straight lines and do not respond to the illusion shown below. They see the lines as of equal length whereas urbanized Zulus have the same trouble as we do in assessing which line is longer than the other. (In fact, they're both the same length.)

Clearly, colour affects our lives in many ways. We all realize

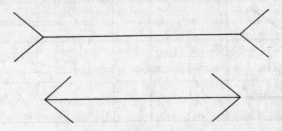

how we 'tune in' to certain colours in our dress, home and work environment but if you think this is a far cry from actually using colours to heal, you'd be wrong because, according to the experts in colour healing, colour is far more important in our lives than simply imparting a 'prettiness' to things.

Unfortunately, like so many of the alternative and fringe medicines, it soon delves deep into metaphysical and spiritual considerations that are very difficult to prove scientifically, so making the whole subject seem cranky. Although colour therapy is a very ancient art, it wasn't until 1933 that a definitive work was published on the subject. *The Spectro Chrometry Encyclopaedia* (in three volumes) written by Dinshah Ghadiali, a Hindu, pointed out that colours represent chemical potencies in higher vibrations. We can explain this in modern terms if we think about the science of spectrometry. Chemical elements burn in a flame to produce a colour specific to each element and it is this fundamental colour that Ghadiali argues is, or should be, the basis of health. He argues that white light contains all the colours of the spectrum in a harmonious balance but that as soon as we alter the body's spectral qualities by adding a chemical of the wrong 'colour' we must expect the body to go out of balance. 'Chemicals are live potencies,' he says, 'their atoms have attractions and repulsions and to endeavour to introduce haphazard inorganic metals into an organic machine is like feeding a baby with steel tacks to make it strong.' Ghadiali describes the construction of lamps, which colours to use and which are suitable for which conditions. He also describes how water or lactose can be charged with colour and then used internally as a medicine.

Light therapy, colour therapy and its close relation gem therapy are all catching on in the USA where several hundred practitioners offer all imaginable variations of therapy in this area. There are about twenty to thirty colour therapists in the UK and probably 100 or so on the continent of Europe. Colour therapy forms an important part of Ayurvedic medicine (see page 114) and is widely practised in India. Although it is still in its infancy in the West, the future looks good for colour therapy provided that more research can be done to prove to western minds that it works.

How does it work?

Colour therapy works somewhat along the same lines as sound therapy (see page 302). First, we have to remember that every living cell is an individual 'battery' of life forces. Just what these forces are, no one knows. They have been called the body's Odic force, have been related to orgone (see page 227) and may be photographed under special conditions by Kirlian photography (see page 211). In sound therapy, sound waves of a specific wavelength are used to so alter the individual cell's (or whole organ's) vibratory pattern as to restore them to health. So, the argument goes, does light or colour restore organs to health.

As we learn more about the nature of matter and realize that matter is really an expression of energy fields, it becomes easier (but by no means simple) to begin to accept that energy itself may be valuable as a healing force. We see how homoeopathic remedies become supercharged with energy during potentization (see page 181) and it is probable that colour therapy acts on much the same lines. In short, shining a blue light on to someone doesn't simply cast a blue colour on to his body but so alters the very functioning of certain of his organs that they can be affected for good or ill. We can all accept the value of the infra-red lamps that we can buy in any local store yet we are loath even to consider that other light colours (wavelengths) might also have healing effects.

The greatest stumbling block seems to be that most of us can't imagine how coloured lights could possibly be perceived by our skin. The fact is that our skin is sensitive to a much greater range of sensations than is generally recognized by western medicine. Research in Russia has shown how easily many people can be trained to feel colours with their fingertips. Some people can even distinguish coloured lights when blindfolded.

That coloured lights do have an effect on the body is easily proven. A study at the New England State Hospital in the USA involved twenty-five normal members of staff with no abnormality of blood pressure. In twenty-five minute sessions during which the subjects were bathed in blue light, a universal fall in blood pressure was noted. When placed in red light the blood pressures all went up. Such an effect was very short-lived, so it didn't constitute a potential cure for high blood pressure but the interesting thing is that by getting the subjects to think about blue they could be made to lower their blood pressures and by having them concentrate on red, to raise them. This is simply another form of biofeedback training but differs inasmuch as the coloured lights actually have an effect in their own right. That this phenomenon is nothing to do with actually seeing the red or blue has since been proved by employing blind subjects who responded in exactly the same way as sighted ones.

How is it done?

A really gifted colour therapist can, simply by looking at the subject, tell what colour he is short of but most people need the help of some simple equipment. An ingenious piece of equipment called a Kilner screen is sometimes used. This consists of two pieces of glass between which a solution of diocene (an indigo-violet coloured fluid) has been poured. This apparently eliminates the coarser ends of the spectrum and enables the viewer to have a more acute view of the patient behind. Experienced colour therapists claim (and there is no way of proving them wrong just as you can't disprove any psychic who says he can see auras as colours around people) they can see auras around the person behind the screen. These auras have colours (just as demonstrated by Kirlian photography) and are altered by rest and activity. The practitioner decides from the patient's medical history and current horoscope readings, which colours he is short of. For example, if a man needed red, he would be lazy, idle, sleepy or anaemic. He might also be constipated or lack appetite.

The great Indian colour healer Jwala Prasada, Mussiff of Benares, makes his diagnosis by the colour of the eyeballs, the nails, the urine and the stools. 'For instance, if a man needs red, his eyes would be bluish, his nails bluish, his urine white and bluish and his excrement white or bluish. Of course it must be remembered that some people want a little red, some more red, while others want a little blue and some more blue and the frequency of doses must be regulated by the degree of want of colour in the system.'

So by a sixth sense, which most of us cannot appreciate, the colour therapist will decide what is needed and how it should be given.

Colour can be given to a patient by many methods and routes. Firstly, white sunlight can be used in a rather non-specific way. We all know how much better we feel when the sun shines and the psychological and physical benefits of reasonable exposure to sunlight are well known and hardly disputed. Colour therapists use sunlight in more controlled ways too and can focus simple sunlight using reflectors and other gadgets so as to expose specific areas of the body selectively. In certain diseases, physical massage with solar-chrome salt bags is advised. This involves a massage with coloured salt-containing cheese cloth bags which have been 'charged up' by placing them in the sun or under a lamp for one hour before the massage.

But it's through the choice of the right foods that colour can work every day of our lives, according to the colour therapists. All vegetable matter has its characteristic colour, as does all inorganic matter. For instance, a person needing red to balance his body healthily will need beetroot (tops and roots), radishes, red cabbage, spinach, aubergines, most deep red skinned fruits, red currants etc. So a colour therapist will, in addition to specific colour treatments, rebalance the body by suggesting the appropriately coloured food. This is based on the assumption that it is no accident that foods are the colours they are and that they contain parallel groups of chemicals and other substances that are essential for health.

Another way that colour therapy is given is as 'rainbow healing'. This is probably the cheapest way of getting colour into the body. Water, if placed in coloured containers and exposed to sunlight, takes on some of the energies of the colour of the container and so can be drunk with benefit by the person short of that colour.

But it's colour breathing that really does most good, according to some therapists. This is really a form of meditation that is best practised on retiring at night or on rising in the morning. According to Roland Hunt in his book *The Seven Keys to Colour Healing*, the subject is 'realizing that Colour is pouring upon him from the sunshine, the very earth, or from the treatment lamp in beneficent radiation, awaiting only his active awareness to become increasingly and permanently beneficial'. A simple affirmation or mantra attuned to the colour being used is often useful, he claims. Hunt finds that the breathing of different coloured light is exhilarating and uplifting and that his subjects feel 'the glow of life and peace of mind'. He feels that colour breathing has a lot more significance than most people would accept and quotes the work of Dr Donald Laird, Professor of Psychology at Colgate University, who confirms that certain bedroom colours cause insomnia and that bright coloured clothes and surroundings had a remarkable effect on backward children.

In addition to harnessing sunlight, manipulating diet and possibly giving internal colour therapy, the colour therapist will use lights of specific colours for very specific conditions. These wavelengths act on the body in well-defined, if ill-understood ways, so as to charge up energy systems in the appropriate body organs or tissues, according to these therapists.

Generally, the patient is either totally bathed in a light of particular colour content or a body part alone may be exposed to the light. The main colour is usually given with a complementary colour (for example green with magenta) which enhances the former's activity. The lights can be used constantly or rhythmically – with differing results. Although there are certain basic rules, each therapist develops his own ways of using colour within this framework.

Does it work?

I personally know of no one who has been successfully treated with colour therapy but great claims are made. Red light has been claimed to cure paralysis in adults and children; orange to dispel small gall-stones and small stones in the kidney (Jwala Prasada claims good results with orange in cholera); diabetes and constipation are said to respond to yellow; ulcers, syphilis, erysipelas, colds, influenza and breast cancer to green; and teething, boils, fevers, inflammation of all kinds, dysentery, colic, jaundice, cuts and burns to blue, and so it goes on.

One colour therapist I know claims good results in personality development, anxiety states and rheumatoid arthritis – the last responding best to rhythmic yellow and violet. He stresses that colour therapy isn't really an alternative medicine as such. It's more a supplement to what conventional doctors have to offer. He also warns of the dangers of do-it-yourself colour therapy because the wrong combination of colours can cause mental and physical upsets.

As with so many of the fringes of medicine it's almost impossible to explain why colour therapy works, if indeed it does. It's very easy to write off a lot of the positive results as simply a psychological improvement that can occur in any case that has done the rounds of the medical profession and arrives as a last resort at the feet of the colour therapist. All medical treatment is empirical and in the face of evidence from colour therapists and their patients we have to accept that it works. How often, how well and for what conditions we probably won't know for years simply because there's so little research of any kind into the subject. In the meantime, it seems unlikely that colour therapy could do any real harm, so it might be worth a try.

Do-In

Definition

A kind of do-it-yourself Shiatsu massage (see page 298).

How does it work?

Do-in (literally, self-stimulation) is a form of acupressure massage that can be done on oneself. Shiatsu massage requires the presence of a masseur but many benefits can be obtained by applying pressure on acupuncture points oneself – in fact many of us unwittingly do just this every day when we rub various parts of our bodies suffering from aches and pains.

Do-in, when properly practised, is a thorough and somewhat disturbing discipline, at least at first. The person doing Do-in may work systematically around the body along several meridians or simply concentrate on certain parts he feels most need attention. Just as with acupuncture itself, Do-in stimulates the meridians and acupuncture points with benefit to internal organs as well as giving local relief from symptoms. Do-in is mainly used prophylactically but may also be used to cure certain specific conditions. A practitioner I know gave me a simple but effective example. If you feel your back is stiff and you'd like to loosen it up, simply pound the inner surfaces of the arches of your feet for thirty seconds. This will loosen up your back and allow you to be more flexible.

All of the oriental practices such as Shiatsu, T'ai Ch'i and Do-in work to harmonize body forces and return them to normal. Almost everything we do in today's world is, in basic biological terms, abnormal. Travelling in cars, working in factories, exposing ourselves to radiation of various kinds and a host of other pursuits in twentieth-century living have all kinds of as yet inexplicable but 'unbalancing' effects on us. We are learning more every day about the problems produced by abnormal vibrations, from sound to those of microwave ovens. Clearly it's impossible to put back the clock and most of us wouldn't want to, but, argue the oriental therapists, we can do something to help redress the balance by re-harmonizing our bodies' energies and forces. It will be a very long time before we can prove them right scientifically but in the meantime they have an enormous amount of experience to go on and millions of satisfied customers in the East today.

Healing

Definition

The use of a human being to alleviate and cure disease.

Background

The art of healing through interpersonal relationships is very old indeed. Hand healing was used in ancient oriental therapy and in the Egyptian temples of healing the priests used their hands. In the Christian Church today we accept the laying on of hands and healing is widely practised by lay people too.

Healing is one of the most difficult fringes of medicine to describe, yet it is probably the most common. There are more people healing in one way or another than there are doctors in any country simply because a lot of paramedical people such as nurses and physiotherapists and many fringe practitioners such as osteopaths and chiropractors as well as doctors are healing every day even if they don't realize they are. Then there are the people who call themselves healers – and there are thousands of those in every western country. Lastly there are the millions of people the world over who seem to have an *ad hoc* healing power but don't even realize they have it.

As we saw in the Introduction, Man is a highly complex creature but in our efforts to bring him down to an understandable level, we seem to have lost sight of a basic fact. Man is *not* simply a very complicated machine, as anyone who has thought deeply about life will bear out.

How can we explain the myriad of so-called miracle cures? Or the death of one spouse immediately following the other? A broken heart? Any doctor will tell of how some patients seem to will themselves dead when they have an illness, whilst others pull through against fearful odds for no apparent reason.

The trouble with attributing cures to any supersensible being or force is that such a force is impossible to measure or even detect and this baffles doctors. Most doctors are not, in fact, working as scientists, yet many like to think of themselves as behaving in a controlled, rational, scientific way. Because the human subject is so infinitely complex, such a cool and calculated approach may not be desirable, necessary or even sought after by the patient.

Pure science and its application come into force when removing an appendix or curing pneumonia, but even with such seemingly clear-cut cases the story is not as simple as it at first seems. There are questions about such an apparently commonplace and simple condition as appendicitis which modern medicine cannot answer.

For many years it has been known that certain physical diseases are inextricably linked to the mind and its function. Today, research is extending this list of so-called psychosomatic diseases to such an extent that it is possible that all disease may soon be linked to the mind or spirit.

There is, for instance, an enormous body of evidence that many cancers are at least in part psychosomatic in origin. This has been remarked on by many distinguished doctors through the ages and, even as early as the second century AD, Galen observed that 'melancholic women are more prone to cancer than are sanguine women'.

Could it be then that the millions of pounds being spent on cancer research each year are being spent on looking at the wrong sorts of things?

The trouble with any cure is that it is impossible to dissociate the psychological effect of the healer as a person from the pure physical or chemical effects of the surgery or the drugs he prescribes. How many times have people been to their doctors and felt better simply because the doctor has reassured them that all is well?

More than 40 per cent of all patients in the average GP's waiting room have no physical ailment that we can detect – it is their flagging spirits that need bolstering and it is here that modern medicine seems to fall so lamentably short.

Healing simply makes use of a sort of empathy as the main source of healing power. If the healer or the patient believes that some sort of supernatural being gives this healing power, it can be called faith healing but the spiritual healers (not to be confused with spiritua*lists* – although some are both) do not demand that their patients believe in anything.

Many healers in the West are practising Christians and attribute their healing powers to the intercession of Jesus Christ but do not necessarily make such demands of those they treat.

Many of the miracles performed by Jesus were possibly a form of faith healing but others again were more akin to spiritual healing because sometimes the cured person had no faith and yet was 'made whole'. Millions of pilgrims to Lourdes and other holy places make their journeys in faith even though they must know that the statistical chance of their being cured is small.

Ironically, one of the greatest single sources of antagonism to spiritual healing today comes, not from medical men, as one would expect, but from the Church. Most formal churches have been unable to endorse spiritual healing, for different reasons, and as a result small bands of spiritual healers formed breakaway churches or religious groups under whose banner they healed the sick.

Nearly all the main churches have now carried out studies into spiritual healing with varying results. There are enough well-documented cases of spontaneous spiritually-induced cures to encourage many clergy but the official line is still a hard one.

In 1956 the British Medical Association published a report on 'Divine Healing and Co-operation between Doctors and Clergy' which said that 'through spiritual healing, recoveries take place that cannot be explained by medical science'.

The power to heal is probably almost universal but healers work in so many different ways that a classification is almost impossible. However it's helpful to consider three different types of healing. Obviously this classification can't be considered anything but tentative and often there is a component of each in any one healing situation.

The first type of healer is typified by the so-called spiritual healer. He works on the principle that whatever one believes can be made to happen. He achieves this by extending the patient's consciousness so that he is more 'in tune' with a higher level of spirituality. He helps get the patient into the supersensible world described in the Introduction. Once the patient is truly in tune with God (or whatever he believes the supersensible force to be), he is open to really remarkable possibilities for cure. Under states of great attunement people actually can experience 'miraculous' cures. Longstanding rheumatic nodules have disappeared within minutes, goitres reduced in size in hours and paralyses and weaknesses dispelled in front of the patients' eyes.

'I get a tremendous pleasure from being able to do the seemingly impossible,' says one leading spiritual healer. But he admits he does not know how it works.

'I feel there is some supernatural life force, that I call God, which uses me as a sort of transformer through which He channels the healing power into the patient. I do not begin to know how it works, but however it happens I do not even need to have physical contact with the patient for it to be effective.'

He then tells of well-documented, instantaneous cures that he has effected on the other side of the world – presumably by a process of thought transference. Who can argue? We only know about what two-tenths of our brain does – who is to say that a part whose function we do not understand might not transfer thoughts to others and receive messages from them?

'Of course, quite a lot of the so-called spiritual healers are very odd,' says the healer. 'Some still go through all sorts of histrionics, rubbing and scrubbing their patients to rid them of all their ills. This really is nonsense. Spiritual healing is a very personal and natural thing. Anyone can do it, we all have the potential. But I think it takes about six to eight years of training to get really good at it.

'Anyone can benefit from it too, although I would not pretend that we will cure everybody of everything. But when you consider we get the flotsam and jetsam of modern medicine, anything we can do is welcome. The most exciting thing to me is that doctors are now beginning to take us seriously and are sending us patients.'

Some spiritual healers and many so-called hand healers claim that they use 'pre-physical' energies or life forces to re-order the life forces of the patient. Spiritual healers the world over maintain that they can harness Life's Universal Healing Force, often by performing specific practices. These include deep breathing, other yoga manoeuvres, the use of holy mantra, Christian prayers and a host of other things. However it is done then, these healers concentrate healing forces in their hands which they then lay on the patient so as to transfer the healing power. The healer is thus a kind of healing force accumulator and does no healing in his own right – he is simply the instrument through which the healing is channelled. Shiatsu (see page 298) is one such healing method and Do-in (see page 151) is a form of do-it-yourself healing.

The second kind of healing (spirit healing) includes contact with the world of disincarnate spirits. Many clairvoyants, spiritualists and similarly psychic people can, they claim, contact other beings and ask their help. Such healers are not conscious of their own action but make a request and receive a mental answer or some outward manifestation. Most of these healers do not have any concept of a 'higher self' yet they can, and do, get results. The healing is said to come not through them but direct to the patient in need.

The last kind of healing is that which is carried out by many doctors, radionics practitioners, homoeopaths and many, many others. This kind is, I suggest, brought about by the power of positive thought. Placebo studies show time and again that anything between 20 and 60 per cent of patients get better when given quite useless tablets but I maintain that the doctor giving them (if he is a healer and genuinely wishes the patient well) imparts a healing pattern to the tablets which then do their job.

We have seen how radionics is thought to work (page 276) along these lines and it is quite possible that many healers work by this same method of thought transfer.

But as well as these three groups of healers there are many others that seem to latch on to psychic phenomena and use these to heal or diagnose illness. Some healers, while asleep, find that their minds leave their bodies and heal other people at a distance. Other healers perceive that particular surroundings are harmful or disease-producing or that illness will arise from a physical object or from a noise.

One group of healers is perhaps especially worthy of mention if only because its members are numerous yet ill understood. Christian Scientists are a sect of orthodox Christians dating from 1879 when Mary Baker Eddy founded the Church of Christ, Scientist. Today there are over 3,500 Christian Science Churches in some fifty-seven countries. Christian Scientists are interesting in the context of healing because they emphasize the importance of drawing closer to God in all healing. Healing, they maintain, is proof of God's care for Man. Faith is a valuable asset but not essential as people who are not Christian Scientists, yet have been cured by them, will testify. Christian Scientists, contrary to popular opinion, are allowed to go to doctors but many choose not to do so, wishing rather to cure themselves by spiritual means which usually means praying and putting their trust completely in God. Even very severe illnesses and broken bones will not take the true Christian Scientist to doctors but as a sect they have nothing against conventional medicine for other people and even occasionally for themselves in extreme situations. What makes Christian Science interesting is that this personal, God-centred, mind over matter healing method really does seem to work. Christian Scientists, according to one of their leaders, live longer and American life insurance companies give them preferential premiums, they're such a good health risk.

So whether it's something you do 'for yourself' or whether it's something that's done 'to you', healing is widely practised and highly successful. But in all these forms of healing, no one for a moment pretends that he himself actually does any of the healing – the healer is only the channel through which God, Life's Universal Force, or whatever it is, acts.

How is it done?

Clearly, as healing methods are so different, the reader will have to refer to particular healing methods outlined in the book under their respective entries but here I'll describe briefly what most people understand by healing – the laying on of hands or hand healing.

> SPIRITUAL HEALING IS A VERY
> PERSONAL AND NATURAL THING. ANYONE
> CAN DO IT, WE ALL HAVE THE POTENTIAL

Each healer has his or her own way of doing things and each acts intuitively. Some healers touch their patients on the head and others on the troubled area. Some healers use their fingers, some the palms of their hands. Others don't even need to touch the patient at all, as we have seen. Absent healing is a well proven phenomenon and possibly works by thought transfer (see Radionics, page 276).

The healer completely relaxes himself and tries to remain as passive as possible so that the healing forces can be active through him. He'll often think of the part of the patient's body that needs help and by doing so channels the healing energies there. The healer's hands may sense heat, cold or pins and needles and there may even be joint sensations. It is at this stage in the healing session that the patient often feels sensations transmitted from the healer and is the stage at which Kirlian photography (see page 211) of the hands shows an enormous increase in the healing aura.

There are no rules as to how quickly any given condition will respond to hand healing. Some conditions take only one session – others many. Very serious conditions may need daily treatments but usually one a fortnight is enough.

But just as this is remarkably effective for many people, so is it very demanding on the healer. He has to be very calm so that nothing gets in the way of the healing process and he may have to spend hours in prayer, meditation, breathing exercises or whatever to keep himself receptive to the healing forces. Healing can be very exhausting for the practitioner and on occasions he may actually get pains himself as he is healing. The patient may become very relaxed or even frankly sleepy and some hand healers advise a period of rest before going back into the hurly burly of life again. A few patients become disturbed emotionally or undergo a psychological catharsis after hand healing.

Does it work?

Harry Edwards, the world famous English spiritual healer, claimed that he failed to cure only 20 per cent of those who came to him. Other healers estimate a 70 per cent cure rate but the most realistic of them claim to help significantly about 50 per cent of those that come to them. This may seem a low success rate but when it is remembered that almost all these patients have exhausted what orthodox medicine has to offer and certainly don't have self-limiting diseases, it is in fact very high.

There is an enormous amount of literature on psychic phenomena, especially in the USA and the USSR, but properly controlled experiments using healing are few and far between: as with most other fringes of medicine, the practitioners are too busy using their skills to conduct research. Healers need medical co-operation (until recently not forthcoming) in order to classify the conditions treated in a way that will satisfy the orthodox medics. One study took twenty-five mice with identical experimentally induced wounds on their backs and compared their healing rate with twenty-five similar mice which were subjected to healing from a professional healer. A further twenty-five mice were subjected to a lamp's heat to simulate exactly the amount of heat given off by the healer's hands during his healing sessions. The twenty-five mice that received healing did in fact make dramatically faster recoveries than those in the other two groups.

Kirlian photography has now opened up new horizons by proving that something is happening in a healer's hands during healing. When a healer is thinking positively about healing, Kirlian photographs of his hands show his body forces change in character to become much more active. His body's energy fields are greatly 'supercharged', especially in his hands.

Although people all over the world know that healing works, it is still poorly regarded by the orthodox scientific and medical world. In the USA, the medical profession and pastors of the church are allowed to heal but lay healers aren't allowed to touch patients. On the continent of Europe there's enormous interest in the subject, especially in Germany, but it is illegal in continental Europe though tacitly tolerated in some countries.

The UK has the most formal set-up for spiritual healing and it is estimated that there are 6,000 or so healers in practice today. There are probably as many or even more in the USA but many are not qualified as are those in the UK and may be working under the guise of other therapies such as mind control. There is, however, an American Spiritual Healers' Federation.

What of the future?

There are those in the fringe medical world who think that healing is in for a period of dramatic growth. Certainly, interest is greater than ever before, notably in the UK where the medical profession is at last beginning to take a serious interest and trials are being started. Given that so many people have the skill to heal and that many more could be developed into good and useful healers, perhaps there is a real future for healing in the West. Healing transcends religious beliefs (which is a bonus in a substantially faithless society as in the West today) and can even work for sceptical patients. Combine this with its cheapness and speed and you have a real power for good in a world increasingly disenchanted with drugs.

Herbal Medicine

Definition

An ancient, worldwide system of medicine using plants to prevent and cure disease.

Background

To the botanist, a herb is any plant that doesn't contain woody fibres (lignin) and so has no persistent parts above the ground. To the medical herbalist, a herb is any plant of medicinal value. There are at least 350,000 known species of plants; the Harvard taxonomic collection contains two and a half million herbarium sheets, yet we've only looked at about 10,000 plants from a medicinal point of view. It would hardly be surprising therefore to find that there are hundreds or even thousands of medicinally valuable plants that we simply know nothing of.

The use of plants to cure disease is older than Man himself. Animals ate plants of certain kinds when they fell ill and indeed they still do. Anyone with a dog will know how it seeks out grasses when it feels off colour but this isn't simply a quirk of domestic animals. Evidence from all over the world shows that animals are naturally drawn to certain plant materials when sick, even if they are substantially carnivorous. So it is with Man. Over his whole history he has evolved along with the plants and animals that surround him. Man has always been dependent on the plant world for his nutritional survival and especially so as three of the fatty acids essential for life (linoleic, linolenic and arachidonic acids) are found almost exclusively in the plant world. In prehistoric times Man slowly built up a bank of knowledge gleaned by trial and error as to which plants were useful in certain ailments.

Ever since records have been kept, there have been herbal medicines. The Chinese had sophisticated pharmacopoeias (lists of useful drugs) in 3000 BC but if the contents of a grave opened in 1963 in Iran are anything to go by, plants were used medicinally as long as 60,000 years ago! The Assyrian King Asurbanipal's library contained a clay tablet listing 250 vegetable drugs dating from 2500 BC and the ancient Egyptians also had a deep knowledge of the subject. Aesculapius, the Greek God of healing, is symbolized by a serpent, because serpents were renowned for their ability to seek out healing plants.

The great growth in herbal remedies came with the development of printing. Early herbals (books of herbal remedies) were, of course, handwritten. This was enormously painstaking and slow which not only retarded progress but meant that few would read the final output – even if they could read. But with the coming of printing the whole scene took on a new dimension. William Caxton printed hundreds of medical textbooks in the fifteenth century and as more people could read and learn about herbalism, interest grew until the publication of probably the greatest work in English on this subject, Nicholas Culpeper's *Complete Herbal*, in 1653. Other books had been written in Latin but this was the first in the vernacular and so available to the average man.

The trouble with much of herbal medicine historically though, and this is true right up to and including the work of Culpeper, was that there was so much magic and myth combined with it. In Renaissance times botanists were doctors and vice versa. As time passed, botanists with a special knowledge of medicinal plants became very powerful and next to the rulers in influence. Many simple traditional herbalists used magic and astrology in combination with plant cures but these practices drew criticism from the Church of Rome which held that such healers with their pagan rites and beliefs had to be stamped out. Witch burning was a logical next step especially as many of these early herbalists knew so much about fertility control and abortion which further annoyed the Church to whom children were sacred. As a result of such persecution, herbalism suffered a considerable loss of prestige and many useful remedies were scarcely used.

The death knell of herbal cures was probably sounded by Paracelsus, the Swiss physician, who lived in the sixteenth century. He and the other 'alchemists' that followed put their faith in inorganic remedies such as mercury and antimony in addition to herbal cures. Although the alchemists were not the first to use inorganic medicines (Ayurvedic physicians had used them thousands of years before), they were probably the first 'moderns' to do so. Paracelsus and his fellow alchemists also used chemistry as a blind to cover their psychological activities which would have led to their being burnt by the Church. This was the birth of the chemical approach to medicine that we live with today. The fashion in drug treatment was to concentrate on inorganics and as a result herbal remedies became quaint oddities.

With the growth of scientific interest in plants, many of the names given by the great Victorian taxonomists of the nineteenth century reflected the plants' medical use but by then inorganic compounds were in their heyday and plant cures used only by a few.

In the eighteenth and nineteenth centuries a herbal tradition emerged from North America as American Indian and European knowledge was pooled. It was in America in the early 1800s that Samuel Thompson started treating people with herbal remedies. The laws of the day (still in force) specifically prohibited the practice of medicine without a degree and he was imprisoned and tried on several occasions. The interesting thing about this episode is that it epitomizes so much of our modern thinking on herbalism. Thompson was condemned because it was claimed he had the nerve to pretend to be able to heal people and that this was highly unlikely because he was a simple man of the soil and therefore couldn't be compared with a gentleman doctor. Herbalism today still carries this very same cross.

The nineteenth century was the heyday for tinctures, potions, cordials, lotions and electuaries and soon exaggerated claims were being made for all kinds of plant extracts and 'patent' medicines. Mandrake was the most widely praised of all, claimed to cure barrenness, plague, induce sleep, relieve pain and restore hair to the bald! One twelfth-century writer claimed it would 'cure every infirmity except death'! Above all though, mandrake was renowned as an aphrodisiac. Partly because of such ridiculously broad claims and partly because of the growth of interest in chemistry and the synthesis of fast-acting powerful drugs at the turn of this century, herbal cures became unfashionable and all but died out in orthodox medical practice. Today's doctors wouldn't consider herbal remedies as such although nearly a third of all pharmaceutical products are derived from plant sources or are synthetic chemical replicas of them.

How does it work?

Herbal remedies were in use long before Christianity and the Ancients believed that when God created the earth he created plants to be of medicinal value to Man. In the seventeenth century it was widely held that God had given us clues as to which plants would cure which diseases and so the Doctrine of Signatures emerged. This stated that plants (or parts of plants) that looked like certain body organs would contain remedies that acted on those organs. Thus the pomegranate was supposed to be good for the blood, wood sorrel for heart trouble, hepatica for liver ailments and so on. But it soon became apparent that had this been God's intention, he hadn't done his homework because there were lots of exceptions to the scheme. There were, for example, many medicinally valuable plants that couldn't by any stretch of the imagination be said to look like any part of the human being. It is possible that the pattern of a plant might have therapeutic value but for more on this see Bach remedies, page 118.

Plant remedies may act in conjunction with astrological forces as was claimed by old medical herbalists but if they do, it is as yet difficult to prove. Certainly Paracelsus and Culpeper thought the time of the month or the time of the day a plant was picked for its medical use was important. We can't as yet prove them right or wrong but the more we learn about plant biochemistry, the more sense there seems to be in their belief. It is now well known that plants are highly dynamic and active things. All through the day chemicals are being made, circulated and reabsorbed elsewhere. This means that there really are best times of the day to pick a plant for the optimum concentration of certain naturally produced chemicals. At certain times any one valuable substance may well be most concentrated in the leaves and at others in the roots. This cycle varies not only day by day but also month by month and certainly with the seasons of the year. There is a vast amount of research yet to be done to find out exactly which chemicals appear in which part of medicinally useful plants and when. Many an unfortunate was burned at the stake as a witch for knowing the answers to these very questions and much of the folklore that might have helped us today has been lost forever. There are enough records for modern science to be able to pick up the threads but the job is an enormous one.

As far as we can tell, the major way in which plants help cure and prevent diseases can be explained on a biochemical basis. The world literature abounds with evidence but it all needs unifying and explaining in modern biochemical terms. The Herb Society in London is going to do just this. It plans to create a computerized data bank of all the learned papers published in hundreds of journals and dozens of languages. But even so the job is a daunting one and there simply aren't enough highly trained plant biochemists to be able to do the necessary new research.

The British Herbal Medicine Association's Scientific Committee has recently published the first volume of a new pharmacopoeia which is now officially recognized by the Department of Health and Social Security. Two more volumes are to be published very soon and the whole task has taken a team of highly qualified botanists ten years to complete.

Drug companies are already screening thousands of potentially useful plant substances, spurred on by the successes of classical herbal medicine and the increasing difficulty of finding new active products. The bactericidal effect of garlic clove oil on typhoid bacilli is twenty-four times greater than that of carbolic acid as measured by the most modern methods, so we're not talking about imaginary properties. The trouble is that naturally occurring medicinal substances seem to be modified by the presence of a host of other natural substances in the plant and this makes the research all the more difficult. Classically, drug research looks for single active substances and either extracts them as they are or creates them in the test tube so that they can be manufactured on a large scale. This may be a fool's paradise though because it leads to the active substance being given on its own. Modern research is showing that plants contain secondary enhancing and/or side-effect-eliminating substances. Take digitalis, for example. This foxglove extract was widely used to cure dropsy (an accumulation of body fluids secondary to heart failure) with very few side-effects. But once the active principle was isolated it was found to be more potent and to produce more side-effects than the natural leaf in the right dose.

In addition to protective and modifying substances in association with useful plant chemicals, there are also ways of modifying frankly poisonous plants to make them valuable to man. Rural African medicine, for example, uses plants widely and has developed clever ways of treating poisonous plants so as to render them inactive in toxic terms yet retain their pharmacological activity. We could learn so much from them. Unfortunately, the size of the task is so great and the current trend for 'pure' chemical-based drugs so powerful that people haven't taken the opportunity to benefit from the experience of herbal practitioners the world over.

One of the problems confronting western minds is that herbal medicines are very difficult to standardize but there again so are

Some common ailments and their suggested herbal remedies

Asthma Aniseed, celandine, elder flower, fennel, hyssop infusion, liquorice root, valerian

Bladder problems Bearberry, birch, chamomile, infusion of chickweed, cowberry

Blood pressure Mistletoe

Boils Chamomile, flax, marjoram, marsh mallow, nasturtium, sanicle, scarlet pimpernel infusions, compress of thyme

Bronchitis Comfrey

Burns Raw onions and potatoes

Colds Tea of agrimony, chamomile inhalations, cinnamon, ginger, marjoram infusions, peppermint, sunflower seed oil, thyme, yarrow

Constipation Alder, blackthorn, fennel, liquorice, molasses, prunes, slippery elm

Coughs Calamint, elder blossom, hyssop, sunflower seed oil

Diarrhoea Infusion of blackberry root, cinnamon

Dyspepsia Caraway

Fatigue Agrimony, marjoram, peppermint, rose hips, yeast tablets

Fevers Tincture of aconite

Flatulence Caraway, tincture of cardamom, charcoal biscuits, fennel, garlic, turmeric

Gout Colchicum, hyssop, juniper

Headache Chamomile, lavender (as cold compress), mint, poppy

Heart disease Foxglove, motherwort

Insomnia Aniseed, bergamot (taken as oswego tea), hops, valerian

Menstrual problems Lady's mantle tea, mistletoe, rose hips

Piles Lesser celandine, plantain (pulped leaves applied locally)

Rheumatism Tonic tea of agrimony, chamomile, cuckoopint externally, ground elder, hyssop, mugwort, onion rubbed on joints, rosemary externally

Sore throat Stinging nettle (gargle)

Sprains and bruises Arnica externally, marjoram oil

Stings and bites Horseradish externally

Stomach ulcers Liquorice

Toothache Oil of cloves, elder (held in mouth), tansy

Unsightly veins Fresh coltsfoot leaves in a poultice, valerian

Vomiting Chamomile, peppermint, spearmint

Wounds Lovage

patients! Different individuals of the same plant species grown in different soils, at different times of the year, harvested on different days and even stored in different ways will all contain different amounts of the active medicinal substance. This was perfectly acceptable when local physicians made up remedies for local people because they would standardize their own preparations. It isn't true today though when large drug companies supply drugs all over the world. This takes us right back to one of the most basic principles of herbal medicine – that a man relates to the plants surrounding *him*. This means that the extracts of plants growing in our own environment are most likely to help cure the conditions we suffer from. There's no reason to believe that we have to go to the Himalayas to gather a rare flower to cure a disease seen in Europe. This theory is being implemented today with allergists recommending asthma and hay fever sufferers to eat local honey so that they will be desensitized to *local* pollens to which they might be allergic. But the pharmaceutical industry can't function if it has to tailor make drugs for localities and small groups of people – so drugs have to be standardized. The major problem with this practice is that people aren't standardized and it's this that has led to disillusion with much modern drug therapy.

What is it used for?

Herbal medicines are not used to cure diseases as such. Herbalists try to choose a remedy that will, from their experience, return the body's balance to normal. However, many herbal medicines relieve symptoms rapidly which the patient sees as a cure. Very acute medical and surgical conditions such as appendicitis and severe pneumonia are unlikely to respond to herbal cures but many practitioners tell of excellent results with very serious medical and surgical conditions if they are caught early enough. Conditions such as these are rare events today though, compared with the great mass of troubles that present to most doctors. Herbal cures seem to produce best results in those suffering from conditions brought about by the imbalances of modern living and will only work really well if the patient alters his life style in such a way as to return to a more natural and healthy way of life. Herbal cures can't work miracles in an overweight, heavy smoker who sleeps badly and takes no exercise.

Over the last 100 years or so (a pinprick in the evolution of Man) we have changed our environment enormously but nowhere more so than in the food we eat. With the movement of people from country into town, the need for mass produced, mass marketed food became great. No longer could people produce for themselves the food they needed – they had to rely on farmers to supply them. This led to the formation of a massive food industry which produced, stored and marketed its wares to the urban millions. So that it could do this and make a profit by doing so, manufacturing processes had to be invented and new methods of food processing, refining, preservation and storage developed. This led to our current food which is liberally laced with large numbers of chemicals quite alien to our bodies. Just read any label on a packet or can to see what I mean.

Unfortunately these chemicals are beginning to have all kinds of unwanted effects on our bodies as our food becomes further removed from its original plant sources and modified by chemicals added either to it or to the growing plants and animals from which it comes. It has taken a long time to realize that we suffer unnecessary illness because of eating quite unnatural foods. When I say 'unnatural', I mean in evolutionary terms. After all, the unprecedented changes in our diet that I am referring to have taken place in eighty to a hundred years, which is a drop in the ocean of the history of Man.

Many conditions seen today in the average doctor's surgery are brought about by this unbalanced and unnatural food we eat and to which we are not adapted. They include illnesses as different as headaches, diarrhoea, ulcers, infections, constipation, stomach aches, asthma, skin rashes, eczema, colds and many, many more. Whether emotive diseases like cancer or multiple sclerosis are caused by poor nutrition, we don't know. There are plenty of other conditions we can do something about so it seems sensible to act on these while researchers look for cures for these more dramatic conditions. Today's herbalist deals almost exclusively with people suffering from conditions produced by the imbalance of man and his plant world. This means that the modern herbalist concerns himself very greatly with food.

How is it done?

The modern qualified herbalist in Britain is not medically trained but does undergo a training lasting several years. When someone goes to see a qualified herbalist he'll be asked to give a complete medical and dietary history, probably dating from birth. This might at first seem strange but if you bear in mind that the whole pattern of a person's allergic potential is set in infancy, you'll probably be amazed. Allergies are seven times less common in children who have been fully breast fed compared with those who are bottle fed and modern research is pointing the way towards an understanding of many adult diseases in terms of breast or bottle feeding. Work under way in the UK is beginning to link heart attacks with bottle feeding in infancy and other diseases such as ulcerative colitis and coeliac disease are commoner in adults who were bottle fed as babies compared with those who were breast fed. The switch from breast to bottle feeding is just one (albeit an important one) of the dietary changes that have occurred in the last 100 years but is just the sort of thing that will be of great interest to a herbalist when taking a history. Once the detailed history has been taken, the herbalist may use modern diagnostic methods such as taking the blood pressure, ordering X-rays or even doing biochemical tests if necessary. Usually though, none of these are required because the good medical herbalist will have arrived at a diagnosis by the end of the history taking stage.

Next comes the treatment. Most good herbalists make their

own remedies from plants or extracts they have bought and blended or even collected themselves. Every patient receives a unique treatment, tailor-made for him. The principle of herbalism is to treat the patient himself and not his disease. There are, of course, some basic remedies which are used time and again for certain conditions but other extracts will be added according to the individual patient's particular problem. Herbalists don't use pain-killers as such or indeed any specific 'anti-anything' compounds – all their remedies stimulate the body's own defences to produce the desired effects. The dosage of all the remedies is very low (though not homoeopathic) so side-effects are very rare indeed. Some of the remedies rather than actually aiming to cure anything will simply boost natural body chemicals that are deficient for some reason.

Most herbalists, however, won't simply give the patient a bottle of the remedy and expect him to go away and carry on living as before. An integral part of herbal medical treatment is a complete reassessment of the patient's diet, life style, exercise, breathing and so on to ensure that the underlying cause of the ailment is tackled at source. Patients receiving herbal remedies usually sense improvement within hours and are very often cured of longstanding symptoms within days.

What of the future?

Herbal medicine is almost certainly due for a revival. People today are increasingly disenchanted with modern drug therapy and are open to new methods of treatment that are closer to Nature. The current trend for herb shampoos and similar proprietary products is a symptom of this movement.

The World Health Organization is now very interested in herbal medicine. The International Federation for the Promotion of Natural Therapies is involved with the World Health Organization in discussions on traditional medicines. Many vast countries still depend on herbal medicines for the health care of millions of their people and this link between a natural therapy organization and the World Health Organization must be a move in the right direction. One thing is becoming evident. No country will be able, or indeed will want, to rely solely on any one system of medicine in the future. The traditional cures of the third world can benefit from the best that western medicine has to offer and vice versa.

There are at last signs that the medical world is beginning to take herbal medicine more seriously. 'Pawpaw Cure Saves London Man' ran the headline of a front page story in the London *Evening Standard* in 1977. The case was that of a kidney transplant patient who developed a post-operative infection which was cured by laying strips of pawpaw across the infected wound. The thirty-one-year-old patient recovered rapidly but died later from other causes. On another occasion UK papers carried stories of heart attack prevention by extracts from the seed of the evening primrose. Drug companies, alerted by the publication of results in the medical journal *Thrombosis Research* are now showing interest in the evening primrose. As long ago as the 1940s a Dutch doctor, Revers, used liquorice to cure peptic ulcers and a large drug company has had a drug based on this in use for years. Over the last twenty years more than a third of a million compounds have been screened by pharmaceutical companies for their potential anti-cancer properties but only twenty or thirty have shown any real promise. One of these is a plant substance, vincristine (an extract from *vinca rosea*, a member of the periwinkle family), now used to treat leukaemia.

There is an enormous proliferation of literature in the herbal medicine world, much of it from Russia where the profit motive is not so important and plants are taken more seriously in medicinal terms. Nobody in Russia or China who knows the subject doubts the value of ginseng for example, yet it is still largely ignored in the West.

The future for herbal medicine lies in a greater acceptance by doctors of the possibility that compound therapies may act better than 'pure', single ones. Almost all herbal remedies are complex mixtures of active ingredients which, if given alone, might have no effect or even possibly ill effects yet when given together seem from experience to produce the best effect. Most herbal medicines are relatively cheap and could be easily standardized (given the same amount of time and resources currently employed in the pharmaceutical industry) so as to produce safe, inexpensive treatments. Unfortunately, research is difficult when it comes to herbal therapies because, as with homoeopathic remedies, each is personalized to the patient. To obtain sufficient numbers of exactly comparable patients so that different herbal and non-herbal remedies could be tested would be almost impossible because, unlike trials done in modern western medicine in which very small numbers of variables are taken into account, the numbers of variables involved with a herbal cure would be enormous.

Probably the final proof lies with the patients themselves who, having frequently gone through all that modern medicine can offer, without a cure, obtain speedy and trouble-free relief with natural, herbal medicines. There is no doubt in my mind that over the next thirty years the pharmaceutical industry will spend a lot more time and money looking at existing herbal cures and trying to find new ones. This shouldn't mean screening more and more plants so as to find even more extracts that can be mimicked in the test tube but I'm afraid it will, because that's all we seem to be able to understand in the West today.

Meanwhile, medical herbalists will continue to practise their age-old and well-proven art and chalk up their successes where modern technology fails.

Homoeopathy

Definition

A system of medicine based on the principles that agents which produce certain signs and symptoms in health also cure those signs and symptoms in disease and that the more a drug is diluted, the more powerful it becomes.

Background

Homoeopathy is not a cranky, way-out type of medicine practised by a handful of odd-ball doctors. There are 300 fully qualified medical doctors practising homoeopathy in the UK and no doubt there are very many more who are not known to the academic bodies. This form of medicine is available under the National Health Service and the Faculty of Homoeopathy in London is recognized in law just like all the other learned medical faculties. Any general practitioner can write a prescription for a homoeopathic remedy and many a local pharmacist stocks homoeopathic medicines. There are also lay homoeopaths who practise successfully in the UK, many of whom combine homoeopathy with naturopathy, radiesthesia, psionic or osteopathic practices.

In 1977 more than 86,000 people went to the outpatients departments of the six homoeopathic hospitals within the National Health Service and no doubt many more went to private practitioners and to general practitioners up and down the country.

Homoeopathy is even more widely practised on the continent of Europe where homoeopathic remedies are mass produced and very popular. South Africa has recently recognized homoeopathy and it is gaining popularity in many other areas of the world in which allopathic medicine is practised. It has always been popular on the Indian sub-continent.

Why then is homoeopathy still regarded by most of the medical profession as being on the fringe and hence probably of little use?

The answer lies basically in the inability of modern doctors to understand how a remedy containing very few molecules (or even none at all) of a healing substance can be active in the body. Modern nuclear science and transistor theory are providing answers to these questions but more of that later. First, how did it all start?

Early in the last century, Dr Samuel Hahnemann, a Leipzig physician, found that when he took cinchona bark, it gave him the same symptoms that patients with malaria suffered. The interesting thing to him was that cinchona bark was currently being used to treat malaria. He thought this so strange that he proceeded to give small doses of medicine to healthy people and himself and carefully noted the effects they produced.

Slowly over the years he built up a list of drugs and the symptoms they produced in normal people and then gave the corresponding drug when a patient presented with that collection of symptoms. He got excellent reproducible results. He found, however, that some patients were made worse by the so-called 'normal' dose of a drug and so started diluting them. He noticed that many actually worked better and didn't produce side-effects in very weak doses.

Since then many doctors and scientists have checked and rechecked Hahnemann's findings and today there are books listing well over 2,000 active homoeopathic substances.

Strangely enough this 'like treating like' principle, now over 150 years old and greatly scoffed at by the medical profession, is seen increasingly in everyday medical practice in various forms. The use of X-rays and radium, themselves a cause of cancer, to cure cancer, is well known. Indeed, certain of the most useful drugs we know today, the heart drug digitalis and the life-saving steroids, are used in clinical situations in which there are symptoms just like the overdosage of these drugs.

Most homoeopathic preparations are extracts of naturally-occurring substances like plants, animal material and natural chemicals. But some are synthetic like other drugs doctors use. In fact the good homoeopath uses ordinary 'allopathic' medicines as well as homoeopathic ones when conditions demand it. Homoeopathic medicines have weird Latin names which, although universally understood, often put people off them. But all in all they're much preferred by patients because they're cheap, almost always taken by mouth, are taste-free, can be stored for long periods without losing their activity and, last but by no means least, never produce toxic side-effects.

Many of us who have been on tablets from the doctor will have thrown more tablets away than we have taken. Many doctors, let alone their patients, are getting alarmed at the enormous misuse and generally adverse effects of drugs today. One study showed that as many as 18·5 per cent of people in hospital were suffering the side-effects of drugs. The interaction of one drug with another is becoming better understood and the more we learn the less we like what we find. On top of all this, drug costs are escalating furiously and much of the bill is paid for drugs that are simply not taken because the patient doesn't get on with them.

How it's done

Firstly, a homoeopathic doctor will take a detailed history, taking into account domestic, personal and psychological as well as frankly medical aspects of the illness. Homoeopathy is 'whole person' medicine. A homoeopath won't just ask you about the symptoms which take you to him and for a very good reason. This is because exactly similar symptoms in you and me will be treated very differently by a homoeopath, depending on a whole host of variables.

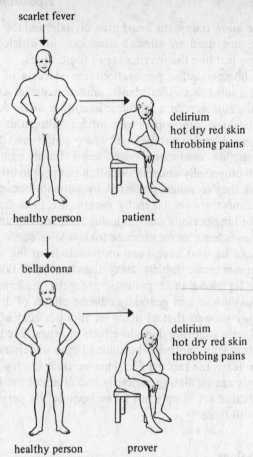

An illustration of the basic homoeopathic principle – 'let like be cured by like'. Belladonna is given because it produces the same signs and symptoms in a healthy person as scarlet fever does in an ill one

In making his diagnosis a homoeopath uses the same tests as other members of the medical profession and of course offers surgery when it's necessary. After all, homoeopathy has little to

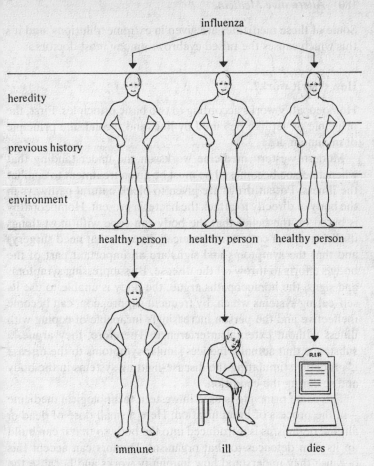

The same disease produces different outcomes depending upon the individual's biological make-up

offer if one's appendix has burst! But when choosing their treatments, homoeopaths take many more factors into account than most ordinary doctors.

Once he's decided on the diagnosis and the treatment required he'll give the smallest effective dose and see how this works.

Some of these medicines are given in extreme 'dilutions' and it's this which causes the raised eyebrows among most doctors.

How does it work?

Homoeopathy works according to two basic principles. First, the principle of 'let like be cured by like' and second, the principle of minimum dose.

Modern western medicine works on the understanding that when a person becomes ill he must be given treatment to combat the illness. Potent drugs are given to block natural pathways in the body or directly to attack the bacteria present. Homoeopathy is based on the belief that the body can cope with most things itself (except of course 'mechanical' illnesses that need surgery) and that the symptoms and signs are an important part of the body's efforts to throw off the disease. By suppressing symptoms and signs, the homoeopaths argue, the body is unable to use its self-curing systems which, by frequent suppression, can become ineffective and the person increasingly incapable of coping with illness without external interference. Therefore, they argue, a substance that actually induces similar symptoms to the disease is probably stimulating the disease-fighting systems in the body and so curing the condition.

This same principle is used in western technological medicine – in the process of immunization. Here a small dose of dead or altered organisms is introduced into the body so that it can build up its own defences to that organism. Doctors can accept this because they understand how immunity works and because the science of antibody formation is well advanced.

But it's when we look at the second principle that real problems occur. When a homoeopath makes up a remedy, he dilutes it with a solid (usually lactose) or a liquid (usually pure alcohol). If a solid is being used as the diluent then the remedy has to be ground up in a bowl to form an intimate mixture with the diluent. This grinding process is known as trituration. A fraction of the mixture is then taken and diluted tenfold (one part of mixture added to nine parts of lactose) and this procedure is repeated.

If the remedy is soluble the same procedure is followed but instead of grinding the spirit with the remedy, the two are shaken vigorously. This is called succussion. The solutions thus produced are called 'potencies'.

The strength of the remedy is expressed as 1c, 2c, 3c etc. as each successive hundredfold dilution and succussion is made. Because this method works in hundreds it is called centesimal as opposed to a parallel method of tenfold dilutions called decimal. In the UK this latter is expressed as 1x, 2x, 3x and on the continent of Europe as 1D, 2D, 3D.

As the remedy is triturated or succussed time after time there comes a stage when there are very few molecules of the original remedy left in the solution. For example by the time 12c is reached there may only be one molecule of the remedy left in the solution yet it would still be homoeopathically effective. The process by which a homoeopathic remedy becomes more and not less powerful as it is serially diluted and succussed is known as 'potentization'.

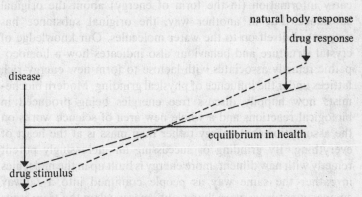

The 'seesaw' of health is returned to normal by giving a homoeopathic drug which may make the person worse before he gets better

Why does it work?

Hahnemann and the many homoeopaths since knew that their remedies worked because their patients had proved it for over 150 years, yet until recently no one knew why. The first thing we have to get straight is that homoeopathic remedies are not active in the molecular chemical sense that ordinary drugs are. The Arndt-Schulz Law expresses the essence of this exactly. 'Large doses of a poisonous substance may prove lethal, smaller doses inhibit, but minimal doses of the same poison can actually stimulate vital cellular function.' This can be demonstrated in the laboratory but why should it be true?

To understand the answer we need to look at the very latest concepts in nuclear physics. Avogadro's Law states that the number of molecules in one gram molecule of substance is $6\cdot023\times10^{-23}$. This means that theoretically if we dilute something to 10^{-24} (that's 1 and 24 '0's . . . i.e. 12c potency) there aren't any of the original molecules left. Recent work has shown, however, that the water in which they were originally dissolved still might carry information (in the form of energy) about the original substance. Put in another way, the original substance has 'imprinted' itself on to the water molecules. Our knowledge of crystal structure and behaviour also indicates how a homoeopathic remedy associates with lactose to form new energy-rich lattices under the influence of physical grinding. Modern biochemists now happily discuss free energies being produced in biological reactions and a whole new area of science works on the assumption that energy rather than mass is at the heart of everything. By grinding or succussing an increasingly potent remedy with new diluent, more energy is built up in the molecules in rather the same way as people crammed into a railway compartment have more 'burst-out' energy when the train stops than a similar number of people sitting in a row of seats.

So the homoeopathic remedy is given to the patient in low concentration but high intrinsic energy state. It is this energy which is then released to stimulate various bioenergetic systems in the body. It has also been suggested by nuclear physicists that such imprinted energy patterns have self-replicating qualities. This would also help explain why homoeopathic remedies work so well – they may actually 'reproduce' in the bioenergetic systems of the body unlike allopathic drugs that, as far as we know, are simply metabolized and excreted.

It may well be that synthetic medicine molecules act in exactly similar ways to homoeopathic remedies in that many of them stimulate basic biochemical pathways at a cellular level. However, most drugs do this in such a relatively non-specific way that they trigger off many unwanted cellular responses in addition to the desired ones. It's rather like using a very long ladder to reach a window. Certainly the modern drug (long ladder) will get you to the window but the long overhang of ladder above the top of the house makes the whole system unstable and potentially dangerous. Homoeopathic remedies are like short ladders that simply gain access to one desired window.

What is it used for?

Homoeopathic remedies can be used for most reversible illnesses, many acute infections but not surgical or corrective procedures. Homoeopathy can't repair a hernia. Early treatment may be recognized by a temporary increase in symptoms (or even the appearance of new ones) before improvement starts. The homoeopathic pharmacopoeia is very flexible, comprehensive and stable compared with the allopathic pharmacopoeia. About twenty remedies can cope with most everyday problems and because they are so safe they are ideal for self-medication and home treatment. Homoeopathic remedies can also be used as preventives and have been used to excellent effect in animals. This is a good answer to those who feel there is a large placebo action with homoeopathic remedies. It's easy to imagine this to be the case in humans but certainly not in a herd of cows!

Does it work?

Undoubtedly the answer must be 'yes'. Millions of people the world over are treated homoeopathically every day. It is a system of medicine with great merit that deserves far greater research effort. This may well come about as pressure on the pharmaceutical industry in the West gets to the point where it is forced to find cheaper yet effective remedies for our ills. There's every reason to believe that homoeopathy could fit this requirement exactly because not only is it effective but it's also safe and cheap.

Unfortunately, it's not easy to prove to sceptics that homoeopathic remedies work because the double blind trial which is held by most doctors to be the final arbiter of a drug's effectiveness either simply can't be carried out at all or can only be done with enormous difficulty. (One such trial has proved homoeopathic remedies superior to standard treatment in a series of burns patients.)

There are all sorts of problems in doing trials of homoeopathic medicines. Usually, if you want to know if a drug is effective in a certain condition, you give randomly allocated patients either the drug under test or a dummy drug. If neither the patient nor the doctor knows which drug is being used (the organizers of the research know but don't see the patients or the doctors during the research) then the effect of the drug can be ascertained accurately and independently. This is the classical 'double blind' trial.

Homoeopathic remedies are so individualized, each one being tailored to the patient himself, that trials like this are at best extremely difficult and at worst impossible. Add to this the fact that the largest homoeopathic hospitals are still very small by normal research standards and you get a situation which doesn't make for easy research. Once again, as with so many alternative therapies, we may not have the resources to produce definitive answers for many years to come. In the meantime, though, we simply have to take results at face value. After all, we're doing it in western medical practice every day.

Hydrotherapy

Definition

The use of water to heal.

Background

The use of bathing as a preventive against and remedy for illness
is very old. Cleopatra is supposed to have bathed in asses' milk
so as to keep her skin beautiful and the Ancients knew that the
human body could be affected by the contents of a bath in which
it was submerged.

It was the Romans who really made bathing for health into a
science and their public baths were beautifully built and decor-
ated, reflecting the large amount of time the bathers spent in
them. Roman baths were rather like a modern hydro or health
farm with all kinds of ancillary facilities as well as the baths
themselves. There were often libraries and gymnasia and sometimes even entertainment for relaxation of the patrons.

Over the centuries bathing in waters with supposed medicinal
properties has become increasingly popular but today finds mass
acceptance only in Germany. Here the state will finance a
person's health cure in a spa on his sickness insurance, much as
it would pay for his other medicines and medical treatments.
France too boasts many spas although water therapy isn't quite
as popular there as in Germany. The UK regards hydrotherapy
as an unnecessary luxury and classes it along with manicure and
other ways of pampering the idle rich. This is unfair because, as
the Germans have found, hydrotherapy benefits everybody and
should by no means be restricted by class or financial barriers.

In the USA hydrotherapy is a popular pursuit but is confined substantially to the rich as in the UK.

What is it?

Hydrotherapy involves the taking of local water by mouth, bathing in it and having other therapies carried out in it. There are many different kinds of healthgiving baths. Cold baths are used in some illnesses but hot baths are more commonly used. Some treatments call for a combination of hot and cold baths alternately. Here are just a few of the therapies that are available in a modern hydro.

Pressure-hosing is a form of water impact therapy. Usually sea water is hosed at the patient under great pressure (he has to hold on to something or he'll fall over, so great is the pressure) from a distance of 25–50 feet. Partly because this is so tiring, albeit invigorating, it is a method little used.

The *salt-rub* involves the hosing down of the patient from a distance of three to five feet with cold tapwater at normal pressure after he has been rubbed all over with salt. Patients say that this leaves them with a sense of well-being.

The *sitz bath* is like a shortened hip-bath so that the patient can sit in it and have his legs completely outside the bath. They are usually in pairs, side by side, one filled with cold and the other with hot water. In front of the cold bath is a basin of hot water and in front of the hot one is a basin of cold. The patient sits in the hot bath with his feet in the cold water basin and then transfers to the cold bath and the hot basin. This is repeated several times and greatly improves the circulation of blood in the legs. Sitz baths are also used for patients with pelvic disorders.

The *Epsom salt bath* induces considerable sweating in the patient. A bathful of water as hot as can be borne has 5–7 lb of commercial magnesium sulphate added to it and is kept topped up with hot water. The patient sweats profusely and gets out to be showered, rubbed down and wrapped in towels to sweat further. After a final warm shower the treatment is complete.

Needle sprays are very fine jets of hot and cold water that are played on to the body with a very invigorating effect. A whirlpool effect can also be produced in a special kind of bath but it is doubtful whether such a bath has any special properties.

The *bubble 'air' bath* is obtained by the massive bubbling up of air through water in which the patient lies. The effect is like a foam bath but with no detergent. This is said to be very relaxing.

Of course the body can be bathed in almost anything. Asses' milk isn't much in vogue today but muds and seaweeds certainly are. Italy and Austria supply the best muds for this purpose.

The most widely used hydrotherapy treatment though is underwater massage. The patient lies in the bath and is 'massaged' by a strong jet of water at 35 lb per square inch pressure. Because the body is submerged it becomes almost weightless and so enables the massaging action of the water to have more effect on the relaxed muscles. This allows more rigorous massage than could be applied in air.

In addition to these and many more, such as Turkish baths, foam baths, scrubbing baths and so on, the patient may also take the water internally as a medicine. Water-only fasts are occasionally used to cleanse the body of toxic substances. Water is also used in colonic irrigation (a procedure in which water is pumped into the colon 'to remove toxic wastes'). Certain yoga practices – the exercise called *nauli*, in particular, involve water. In this, the yogi squats in a bath or stream and by creating a considerable negative pressure in his abdominal cavity, draws up water into his bowel. He then discharges it along with all the waste and toxins.

How does it work?

Water is essential to Man – in fact two thirds of our bodies are made up of water. We can go for weeks without food but can only last days without water.

It is possible that certain waters worldwide at spas, hot springs and hydros do indeed have valuable bio-chemical properties in terms of the chemicals contained in the water. We saw how water can contain memories of substances with which it has been in contact in the section on homoeopathy (see page 182) and it is possible that water under certain conditions in spas and hydros contains such healing 'memories'. Kirlian photography has shown how water mentally 'charged' by a healer has a much richer energy field around it than ordinary water, so perhaps the healing aura of the hydrotherapist too alters the water being used.

Most often though I feel water therapy is beneficial because it is carried out by pleasant, caring people who, together with the pampered atmosphere usually surrounding the therapy, induce a sense of mental well-being in the patient. He then relaxes more and this, coupled with sensible eating, sleeping, drinking and exercise at the hydro, really does make him feel better. The mental improvement in turn produces a reduction in anxiety and stress-orientated symptoms and signs and he goes away feeling better – which is what all medicine is about.

Hypnosis

Definition

The art by which a hypnotist induces a trance-like state of compliance and heightened suggestibility in another person. Contrary to popular belief, almost everybody is susceptible to hypnosis. Indeed, the more intelligent the person, the better he or she responds. It used to be thought that simple-minded, easily influenced subjects were easiest to hypnotize but this has now been disproved. By and large it's easier to hypnotize a willing subject but sceptical or unwilling people can be hypnotized, albeit with greater difficulty.

Background

Historically, hypnosis dates back to the Greeks who used it as a form of therapy for anxiety and hysterical states. In fact these very conditions are still treated with hypnosis today. The ancient Druids called it 'magic sleep' and used it to cure warts and cast spells.

But it wasn't until the 1760s that hypnosis became widely known to the public in Europe. The man responsible for its growth in popularity was Franz Anton Mesmer who used hypnosis to cure patients but in so doing gave the subject something of a bad name because of his theatrical approach. He conducted public demonstrations of hypnosis with very susceptible subjects in deep trance states and made them behave like automatons – much to everyone's amusement.

Mesmer called hypnosis 'animal magnetism' and was convinced that all illnesses were caused by imbalances in this 'animal magnetism'. He did, in fact, get dramatic improvements in many of his patients using these histrionic methods but these were probably people with psychosomatic ailments that were cured by the suggestion and magic surrounding the public demonstrations.

But because scientists of the day couldn't prove there was anything in his methods and because the histrionics were somewhat 'unprofessional' medically and scientifically, Mesmer was ridiculed and lampooned and hypnosis has retained an image of quackery ever since.

Traditional medical circles ignored hypnosis as a useful tool until about 100 years ago when James Braid, nineteenth-century Manchester surgeon, who coined the term hypnosis (from the Greek, *hypnos*, sleep), used it medically, even for major surgery. But after this flurry of interest, mainstream medicine, which remembered Mesmerism and all its connotations only too well, did little to further the art. The British Medical Association looked into the whole subject at the beginning of this century to see if there was a place for it in modern medicine but the findings were not rosy and led to the resignation of the professor of Medicine of University College Hospital in London, a prominent hypnotist of the day.

What is it?

Hypnosis is an altered state of mind but it is *not* sleep. Modern studies using electroencephalography to look at brain rhythm patterns show categorically that a hypnotized subject is neither awake nor asleep. The state is somewhere in between. It is no magic state but simply an altered type of consciousness brought about by the voice of the hypnotist which is persuasive, dogmatic and confident. The subject gets to the stage when she believes that what she is told will happen, will happen – and it usually does. I say 'she' as women are often better subjects than men simply because they are less afraid of letting themselves go. People often ask how they can tell whether they'd be a good subject or not. There are two simple ways of finding out. First ask yourself if you can get 'lost' easily in a book or TV programme. If you readily enter the world you're reading about or watching, the chances are you'd be a good subject. The other test involves a small piece of equipment you can make yourself. Take a piece of thread and hang something from its end so as to form a simple pendulum. Start off with it very still and then 'will' it to do something. If it does what you want it to do this too indicates that you'd make a good hypnotic subject.

One leading hypnotist maintains that single-minded people who can easily concentrate on one thing are his best subjects. People whose minds are very active and questioning tend to do badly. It's nothing to do with being sceptical – some very sceptical but nevertheless susceptible people have been hypnotized with success.

How is it done?

Depending on the reason for which the hypnosis is being used, the methods vary but generally it consists of the hypnotist (who is either medically trained or not) talking to the patient (or subject) in a slow, controlled, persuasive and dogmatic way. It helps if the whole procedure is carried out in a room without distractions but hypnosis can be, and is, done in the hurly-burly of the fairground too. Some hypnotists get their patients to concentrate on an image of some kind. Sometimes they use a light, sometimes a revolving wheel and sometimes they simply ask the patient to imagine something. One medical hypnotist I know always asks people if there is anything that frightens them or upsets them. He took to doing this after asking one patient to concentrate on a garden only to find the man in a full blown attack of hay fever, sneezing furiously and with running eyes!

Basically, the idea behind this type of trance induction is to get the eye muscles fatigued so that they involuntarily close the eyes. The therapist then talks to the subject in a slow monotonous voice as he goes through the stages of induction. All but about

10 per cent of people can be hypnotized quite satisfactorily and about 5 per cent will readily go into very deep trance states and behave in the dramatic way that Mesmer so enjoyed. Some hypnotists don't use any effects at all but simply talk to their subjects.

In the early stages the subject closes his eyes and relaxes. Eighty per cent of people will go into this phase easily. The second stage is a light trance in which the subject can perform simple movements (such as raising an arm) when asked to do so. Stages three and four are deeper and enable the patient to carry out post-hypnotic suggestions. A complete loss of pain sensation is possible in this phase and it is this which enables surgery to be carried out under hypnosis. Even quite major surgical procedures such as amputations have been safely performed under hypnosis.

Bringing a person out of a trance is quicker than putting him into one. After a deep trance during which the hypnotist has made a suggestion (such as 'when I put my hand into my pocket you will stand up') the patient will quite naturally get up at the given signal. The remarkable thing is that when challenged as to why he suddenly got up, the patient will have a perfectly rational explanation. Finally, the patient has to be taken back into a trance state and the post-hypnotic suggestions removed. At this stage the hypnotist ensures that the patient knows he will be quite normal and relaxed on waking. Getting patients into a deep trance state can take a lot of time, so to cut short the proceedings some experienced hypnotherapists train their patients to go quickly into a deep trance state at a pre-arranged signal.

Today the histrionics have disappeared from hypnosis although very occasionally demonstrations on television or at medical meetings still show the more dramatic side of the art. For instance, a girl recently thrust her hand into a bucket of iced water at one such demonstration and had to remove it after thirty seconds because she couldn't bear the pain. Yet under deep hypnosis she was able to keep her hand in the water for half an hour because she had been told by the hypnotist that the water was warm.

But the most remarkable outcome of this experiment was that the level of cortisol (the body's chemical response to stress) in her blood stream was not raised when she was under hypnosis but was high with her hand in the iced water without hypnosis. This clearly shows that the mind has an uncanny control over the body at a level far deeper than most of us would ever imagine.

Another example of the power of hypnosis can be seen as the hypnotized subject is made to regress in time. A hypnotist can make a subject go back through his life to childhood and even to infancy. This is accompanied by almost perfect recall of childhood events in the post-hypnotic state. Sometimes, patients actually talk like children when they are in this state of age regression.

An amazing experiment demonstrates this even more dramatically. The reflex movement of the big toe when the sole of the foot is stroked is normally downwards in people over six months old. Before six months the toe goes up. In patients who have been age-regressed hypnotically, this reflex changes from going down to going up. This is just one of the strange things about hypnosis – it seems to enable the subject to do things he otherwise couldn't possibly do or indeed have any control over.

'This is the sort of thing that most worries people,' says a leading medical hypnotist. 'Patients think they're going to be taken over and made to do extraordinary things. Nothing could be further from the truth. We don't get people to do strange or meaningless things any more. These days, hypnotherapy is used as part of a whole treatment which involves making an accurate medical diagnosis and using it with surgery or drug therapy.'

But although much of this might sound dramatic, the enormous growth in popularity that hypnosis has enjoyed among members of the medical profession is because it works in many conditions where drugs are of little value.

What is it used for?

Hypnosis is basically used in three main areas today. The first of these is for entertainment. Slick professional hypnotists can produce amazing results in subjects in front of an audience. This can indeed be very entertaining. One such international performer reckons to have hypnotized more than 100,000 people in clubs and theatres the world over. But many people are concerned about this use of hypnosis and their concern led to a law being passed in 1953 in Britain that forbade anyone under the age of twenty-one being used in stage hypnosis. Even the seasoned performer I've referred to admits to one accident in which one of his subjects walked straight through a plate glass door but he can only recall three or four incidents of this kind in his vast experience of hypnosis.

The main thing that concerns people about such public demonstrations is that the subjects might be made to do things they might otherwise not normally do. For example it might, they argue, be possible to get a girl from the audience to do a striptease against her will. The hypnotist entertainers say this is unlikely to happen in practice because the very short time the subject is available to them means that they can't exert such a powerful control over her. Research in several countries under controlled laboratory conditions has shown this not to be the case, however. So stage hypnosis remains under a professional cloud in all but the most responsible of hands.

Another modern use of hypnosis is in memory recall. The Los Angeles Police Department is training police from all over the USA and Canada to use hypnosis to help the police themselves and their witnesses to remember things they think they have forgotten. They hypnotize the witness and then get him to re-live the scene of the crime. It's amazing how these witnesses can recall the most incredible detail and this is now leading to the serious use of hypnosis in police work. Police in the UK though are declining to use it because they fear that suggestions made to a witness whilst under hypnosis could be prejudicial to the case.

But by far the greatest number of people are hypnotized for medical reasons and there are many conditions that respond well.

Just as in ancient times, hypnosis still works most efficiently in anxiety and hysteria, but today research is widening the hypnotherapist's scope and asthma, insomnia and many phobias are also commonly treated with great success. Habits like smoking frequently respond and fears of heights, air travel, dentistry and many others are treatable by slow, controlled deconditioning under hypnosis. The more serious addictions like alcoholism and drug habituation don't respond so well because there's a considerable biochemical problem to be overcome in these cases – it's not simply all in the mind.

'I usually try and train my patients so that they can hypnotize themselves,' says a medical hypnotherapist. 'I see patients about once a week for six to eight weeks by which time they're usually much better. After this sort of period they've got the idea pretty well and can put themselves into a trance state and so overcome their problems. I get especially good results with asthma. I train my patients to control their breathing under self hypnosis and this stops the asthmatic attack.'

Very few doctors practise hypnosis on a full-time basis because they feel that it should only be a part of their total medical treatment of a case. Most hypnotherapists are ordinary practising doctors who use the technique as an adjunct to their normal therapy, often using drugs or surgery in parallel with hypnosis.

The dangers of going to a lay hypnotherapist, and there are many of them, are much the same as with going to lay practitioners of any paramedical art or science, namely that they may well persevere with their particular form of treatment on the basis of a wrong diagnosis and may simply not know when to stop. For this reason it's probably wise to try and find a doctor who practises hypnosis or indeed any of the branches of fringe medicine discussed in this book if you want to be safe and sure.

The three most publicized medical uses of hypnosis seem to be anaesthesia (for surgery and dentistry), the control of pain in childbirth and for stopping smoking.

Many dentists that use hypnosis use it to calm phobic patients and to induce a pain-free state in which to operate. Some surgical operations are carried out under hypnosis but they are very few in number because conventional anaesthesia is so quick and safe today and doesn't require the presence of the patient's own hypnotherapist. Modern anaesthesia is also more certain. If you are running a busy operating theatre you can't spend time waiting around because a particular patient isn't responding to hypnosis. Modern chemical anaesthetics are more reliable and this is why they win hands down compared with hypnosis.

The unreliability and the fact that a hypnotherapist is needed there all the time are the greatest drawbacks to the use of hypnosis as a help in childbirth. Hypnosis involves a very personal relationship between the therapist and his patient which means that the specific therapist (and not just any anaesthetist) has to be available at a moment's notice and for long periods once labour begins. This is time consuming and often difficult to achieve, unless the therapist also happens to be the obstetrician (or as is the case in one London teaching hospital – the midwife).

Now to smoking. With lung cancer the biggest cancer killer among men in the western world and a fast growing problem in women, anything that can be done to prevent people smoking must be looked at carefully. Hypnosis does seem to have something to offer here. Official figures are depressing because they define a person as having kicked the habit if he doesn't smoke for a year after the therapy. About 20 per cent of smokers are still not smoking one year after *any* therapy – so can hypnosis improve on this? Many individual practitioners claim the answer is undoubtedly 'yes' and one survey in the North of England found that a method using TV hypnosis was fairly successful. Forty-four of the subjects had completely stopped at three months, another 44 per cent had cut down and only 12 per cent reported no effect at all. If these figures can be kept up for a year it looks as though this method of TV-administered hypnosis could be a hope for the future.

So what of the future? Of all the fringes of medicine hypnosis is probably one of the most acceptable. The British Society of Medical and Dental Hypnosis with a membership of more than 1,000 meets regularly in one of the country's leading medical institutions and sponsors excellent research.

There's also a willingness among hypnotherapists to be subject to scrutiny and independent scientific investigations. In proper hands there is no danger involved in hypnosis and we're moving into an era of medicine in which doctors and patients alike are becoming disenchanted with many drug treatments which don't necessarily cure yet may produce unpleasant side-effects.

For a host of psychological and physical abnormalities, hypno-therapy offers a safe, quick and acceptable cure. After a poor start and a chequered history, hypnosis is undoubtedly here to stay.

Macrobiotics

Definition

A philosophy of life originating from Japan that involves taking a very wide (macro) view of life (biotics). It is a kind of non-religious religion.

Background

Macrobiotics (though not under this name) probably dates back to ancient Greece when it was widely practised as a way to health and happiness through an understanding of Man and the cosmos. But macrobiotics as we know it today is based on the contrasting yet complementary principles of yin and yang. Many of the basic principles of macrobiotics have been practised in most cultures for thousands of years but today we think of it as an extension of our recent interest in oriental religions and philosophies. This is partly because of the work of one man, George Ohsawa, a Japanese who cured his own tuberculosis using methods based on traditional oriental medicine. George Ohsawa started a centre for his teaching in Hiyoshi, Japan, where he taught between 1946 and 1952. In 1952 he began a world tour and visited Africa, India, France, Belgium and other European countries, preaching the gospel of a unifying principle underlying the problem of health. He also visited America to conduct seminars. Macrobiotic summer camps, stores and restaurants soon began to open. His pioneering work was taken up by many people but is probably being pursued and furthered most vigorously by Michio Kushi and his colleagues in New England.

What is it?

As a somewhat global, semi-religious pursuit, macrobiotics is difficult to explain and varies somewhat in its interpretation according to the ability and expectations of the person practising it. It is not simply a way of healthy eating (which is how many people see it); it is not simply a kind of alternative medicine; but it is an intuitive way of living one's life so as to remain healthy and happy. Over the centuries, most countries have lost this intuitive and native instinct as to the right and wrong way to eat and behave generally, according to the followers of macrobiotics and so we are all suffering from unnecessary social, physical and mental ills.

How is it done?

Macrobiotics is a personal philosophy involving wholesome behaviour and eating. Food is considered to be central to life and is thus chosen with great care. The principles of yin and yang – the theory of antagonistic but complementary opposites – govern what foods one should eat. Yin and yang enable us to choose foods that are broadly suitable without having to be slaves to vitamin and caloric charts. Very simply, yin foods include drinks and fruits, food with sweet, sour or hot flavours, those with a large open texture and those which are green, blue or purple in colour. Yin is said to be feminine and yang, masculine. Yang foods are animal foods, cereals and a few vegetables. They are mostly hard or dense and red, orange or yellow in colour.

All foods acquire a quality of yin or yang because of their inherent properties, their speed of growth, their climatic preferences and a host of other variables. So with some considerable patience and care all foods can be classified as yin or yang. Followers of macrobiotics maintain that all disease is caused by an imbalance of yin and yang in the body and a macrobiotic diagnosis soon reveals which type of food is necessary to redress the imbalance.

As cereal grains contain an excellent balance of both yin and yang, they form a very basic part of macrobiotic diets. Many people eating such a diet will aim at eating half of all their daily food as grains, presented in one form or another. Macrobiotic diagnosis is based on the outward appearance of the body and uses signs such as the shape and colour of the body, the colour of the complexion and the state of the acupuncture pulses (see also page 76). By diagnosing whether the body has too much or too little yin or yang the person can redress the imbalance himself by altering his food. Followers of macrobiotics hold that all disease comes from within and not from without as western doctors believe. When a person becomes ill, they suggest he should look into himself to see how he is abusing his body by eating bad food, working in poor conditions, sleeping badly, being too angry or having a negative outlook on life.

Food has vastly more significance than to the average westerner who sees it simply as providing building blocks for his body. Macrobiotics teaches that all foods have their own character and should be eaten by those who share their environment. Because of cosmological and astrological factors that are well understood by much of oriental religion and philosophy, foods that grow in the tropics, for example, are very different from foods that grow in temperate zones. This makes the former unsuitable for people living in the latter.

Because of this reverence for food, great stress is put on the proper cooking and preparation of food. All foods should be chosen from natural organic products growing in the same climatic region and in the same season. Thus there are foods which are best eaten in winter and others that are more appropriate for summer. All foods should be alive until they're cooked (this at first sounds horrific but macrobiotics involves the eating of very little meat, though some fish and dairy products are eaten). Historically ancient species of plants should be cooked more and more recent species less. Foods are only mixed during cooking and are generally discouraged by all reasonable means from losing their unique character and properties. Macrobiotic cooking is a skill but with the wide availability today of the right kinds of foods in health food stores, it is by no means impossible and is bound to produce better food than the average westerner eats.

Processed foods are not used and liquids are kept to a minimum. Local foods are preferred because they're likely to be fresher, contain fewer preservatives and have an affinity for the people living in the area.

Macrobiotics followers are not food cranks but see healthy eating as the main way back to a healthier way of life. Many of them find that once they have been on this type of diet for some time they begin to question their previously held views on work, morality and so on and eventually try for a more wholesome and balanced life in broader terms than food.

Macrobiotics varies considerably from place to place around the world to take account of different people, climates, tastes and expectations but the end point should always be the same – a person who is free from illness, doesn't worry, is full of vitality, sleeps well and loves life.

Does it work?

It is impossible for me to judge macrobiotics on a philosophical or religious plane. From a medical and nutritional point of view it has much to recommend it but is unlikely to catch on in a big way because the mass of westerners are lazy when it comes to food and are loath to spend time preparing good food well. Undoubtedly a macrobiotic diet is a healthy one, especially if it is broadly based and not excessively restricted. Some macrobiotics followers are carried away with enthusiasm and become ill by eating far too few foods. It is thus possible to be deficient in Vitamin B_{12} but this can be remedied by taking the vitamin as tablets if necessary. To be fair though this is a complication seen only in the most fanatical macrobiotics followers as most of them prevent B_{12} deficiency by eating seaweed and certain fermented foods which are rich in the vitamin.

The goal of every child being brought up to eat wholesome, well prepared foods is a thoroughly reasonable one and if macrobiotics can become a way of healthy eating which then provides the person with improved health, he can spend more time enjoying the other things life has to offer. Finally, followers of macrobiotic diets seem to live longer. As we learn more about food everything points to macrobiotics being the way to go. We in the West eat too much protein, too little cereal fibre, too many refined foods, too much sugar and too much of everything. Macrobiotics puts this right and will in my opinion have even more to offer in the future as we become disenchanted with our western processed foods. As for the philosophical and 'religious' side of macrobiotics, people will continue to take it or leave it while availing themselves of its good dietary advice.

Megavitamin Therapy

Definition

A branch of medical and non-medical practice maintaining that we may be deficient in certain vitamins and that the way to make good the deficit and so prevent and cure disease is to ingest very large doses of these deficient vitamins.

Background

Megavitamin therapy is a relatively recent addition to the fringes of medicine. Dr Linus Pauling, double Nobel Prize winner and champion of Vitamin C, was one of the first people to take a serious interest in the effects of large (previously unthought of) doses of vitamins to prevent and cure disease. In 1968 he coined the term 'orthomolecular' medicine from ortho – optimum or best. His early work was centred around the use of Vitamin C to prevent and cure the common cold but subsequent research into the use of massive doses of Vitamin C is confused as to just how valuable it actually is. This debate will no doubt continue for years.

But the common cold is not the only area in which the megavitamin therapists have been active. They have cast their net wide and now claim cures for alcoholism, hyperactive children, certain drug addictions, osteoarthritis, 'neuritis', schizophrenia, depression and other psychiatric disorders. Orthomolecular psychiatry has in fact now taken over as the main focal point in orthomolecular medicine, mainly because the public is tempted by a relatively easy way out of unpleasant diseases and because the alternatives (psychoanalytic therapy or admission to a public mental hospital) are too expensive or unacceptable for other reasons. The thought that one might be able to take a simple vitamin tablet to cure one's schizophrenia is tempting indeed.

The originators of orthomolecular psychiatry suggest that by varying the concentrations of substances normally present in the human body we may help control mental disease. According to their theories, various cells in the body need very different nutrients. Brain and nerve cells need very much more Vitamin B and Vitamin C, for example, than other parts of the body. In short, they maintain that much psychiatric illness is explicable in exactly the same way as is other illness – that is by understanding disordered biochemistry. This is very heartening in many ways because in the UK, for example, the psychiatric establishment is unwilling to accept that schizophrenia is a biochemically related disease. Rather they see it as a family and interpersonal relationship problem. This is deeply disturbing to the parents of a schizophrenic and probably ignores much good evidence that points to actual biochemical abnormalities and deficiencies in at least some of these unfortunate people.

In the USA, however, the pendulum seems, if anything, to have swung the other way – at least in the eyes of the orthomolecular psychiatrists – who now maintain that much mental disease is caused by vitamin 'dependency' states, as they call them, and is thus curable by replacement vitamin therapy. Dr Hoffer, one of the pioneers in the field of orthomolecular psychiatry, suggests that there are two types of vitamin shortage in humans. One is what most of us would call vitamin deficiency and is seen in diseases such as scurvy and pellagra. In these conditions, the addition of normal doses of the vitamin to the diet rectifies and prevents further recurrence of the disease (after perhaps an initial booster dose). 'Dependency' states are quite another matter, he argues. These vitamin diseases are caused because the person can't absorb or otherwise metabolize the perfectly adequate doses of the vitamin that he is getting in his food. He suggests therefore that such patients need very large doses in order that *some* at least gets through to the blood stream after ingestion. There is evidence that the gut is abnormal in many more diseases than we ever thought. Schizophrenia, for example, is accompanied by gut lining changes that are similar to those seen in coeliac disease and coeliacs are routinely given vitamin supplements because it has been shown that they absorb vitamins very badly. It could be that any condition in which the bowel lining is changed means that the patient needs much larger than normal doses of vitamins.

For the brain to function properly it needs the vitamins riboflavine, nicotinamide, pyridoxine, cyanocobalamine, ascorbic acid and folic acid at least. There are other chemical substances that are essential for the healthy functioning of the brain and we have only scratched the surface of brain biochemistry.

The argument goes that the amounts of these valuable substances we absorb from the food we eat may not be optimal and that even many of the minimum daily requirements for these vitamins, as laid down by Government nutrition advisers, are simply much too low. So, claim these psychiatrists, we may need to 'overdose' the body considerably with certain vitamins.

The most recent moves are towards the addition of many vitamins and minerals to the diets of people with these psychiatric diseases; but the main vitamins used are B_3 and C. Nicotinamide (Vitamin B_3) cures pellagra and some psychotic illness. Hoffer and Osmond, the two pioneers in the orthomolecular psychiatry field, recommend a 3,000 mg daily dose of this vitamin when the normal daily recommended dose is 20 mg. It is claimed that even at such enormous doses there is no danger. Vitamin C is similarly used in large doses.

So much for the theory. Scores of 'trials' have taken place on megavitamin therapy – the vast majority in the USA. Dr Russell F. Smith, alcoholism expert of Brighton Hospital, Detroit, claimed a 77 per cent recovery rate in a two-year study of 507 alcoholics treated with massive doses of Vitamin B. At the end of the study, 474 of the 507 patients were looked at. Of these, the 138 who were in 'excellent' shape at the end of the first year after treatment were still in excellent health and had suffered no relapses. Of the 'good' result group, 233 were continually sober and were moved up to the 'excellent' category.

At his clinic in Manhasset, New York, Dr David Hawkins has had some amazing results in the treatment of schizophrenia and alcoholism. The clinic has treated over 4,000 patients, of whom 600 were alcoholic. A study by the American Schizophrenia Association in 1977 found that these 'new' orthomolecular methods had cut the cost of treating schizophrenics by 90 per cent. This clinic was using Vitamin B_3 and Vitamin C in doses of 4,000 mg daily and 50 mg of Vitamin B_6 were also given. Some cases also received 400 mg of Vitamin E daily. No ill effects were reported in any cases – even on such massive doses.

The pioneer of the orthomolecular treatment of schizophrenia is Dr Abram Hoffer who now has 2,000 case records of people treated with massive doses of vitamins alone. Two Californian physicians have been treating a variety of conditions with large doses of Vitamin E. They have used it for intractable skin conditions, night cramps and 'restless legs'.

And so it goes on. Whole books have been written about the value of megavitamin therapy for these diseases and many studies report excellent results.

Does it work?

It's tempting to think that all the reports are valid and that a cure for diseases like alcoholism, schizophrenia, other mental illnesses, drug addiction and overactive children is just around the corner. Alcoholism substantially alters the lives of an estimated nine million Americans; half of all US hospital beds are occupied by patients with emotional diseases and half of these are schizophrenics; possibly as many as 30–40 per cent of American primary schoolchildren are suffering the reversible effects of nutritionally related learning handicaps (according to Dr Charles Edwards, ex-Commissioner, Food and Drug Administration); and the common cold causes millions of lost workdays throughout the western world. It's hardly surprising then that we should look for a simple explanation of these problems and grasp it as *the* answer.

Unfortunately, this is exactly what has happened. In fact, so widespread was the public hope for such cures that an independent Task Force set up by the American Psychiatric Association in 1974 to look into megavitamin therapy called the massive publicity surrounding the subject 'deplorable'.

Most biochemists and psychiatrists refuse to accept that there is any real justification for prescribing massive doses of vitamins – mainly because there is so little convincing evidence. As very few controlled clinical trials have been done with single vitamins, it is difficult to assess what they have to offer. One was done by the American Psychiatric Association with Vitamin B_3 for schizophrenia but showed it to be of little value.

However, in 1974 the Alberta College of Physicians set up a commission of three scientists to look into the whole question after an angry public debate. They reviewed the world literature, talked to all the leading practitioners and heard from patients who claimed to have been cured. The report of this study was reviewed in the *Canadian Medical Association Journal* in 1977 and stated that the three experts were unable to reach any firm conclusions. There was no hard evidence that megavitamin therapy worked but some individual case reports did seem difficult to dismiss. They stressed the need for controlled clinical trials of the treatment of conditions such as schizophrenia, arthritis, depression and hyperactivity in children but were concerned about the possible side-effects of very high doses of vitamins, especially of Vitamins A and D which are known to be toxic in easily ingestible doses.

Shaywitz and his Yale University colleagues, who recently reported a case of a boy with severe Vitamin A overdose, are concerned about this potential overdose, as 10 per cent of children with minimal brain dysfunction referred to their neurology clinic were receiving megavitamin therapy, often from self-appointed nutrition 'experts'. So emotive is the whole subject that the case of this little boy drew two editorials in the influential *Journal of the American Medical Association* in the *same* issue. One referred to the 'murky business of megavitamin therapy in the treatment of learning disability, autism and schizophrenia' and went on to condemn the selling of multivitamin preparations containing '8,000 per cent, 16,000 per cent and 32,000 per cent of the US recommended daily allowance of the B vitamins and Vitamin D'.

The other leader went on to say that classic examples of vitamin misuse are massive doses of Vitamin A for osteoarthritis and neuropsychiatric disorders; Vitamin D for bone thinning; Vitamin C for the prevention of colds; Vitamin B for 'neuritis'; and Vitamin E for sterility and coronary heart disease.

THE COMMON COLD CAUSES MILLIONS OF LOST WORKDAYS THROUGHOUT THE WESTERN WORLD

Most megavitamin therapists don't allow their patients to take harmful doses such as those of concern to these writers and I'm sure that vast numbers of people in the West are in short supply of certain vitamins, trace elements and minerals. The average western refined diet is so poor that it can't hope to supply us with what we need for optimal health. What is needed is a serious controlled trial to examine each area in which megavitamins have been claimed to work. Trials such as the one by the American Psychiatric Association are fine as far as they go but have only looked at a single vitamin. We know from the way herbal remedies act that it is possible that substances working together have more value than exactly the same substances given alone. Too little serious, laboratory-based research has been done as yet in the USA (or indeed elsewhere) to be able to form a definitive opinion on this therapy. Rather than getting over-enthusiastic about a series, however large, of anecdotal successes, scientists need to do extremely detailed (and costly) biochemical profiles in the patient they're about to dose with megavitamins.

I know this is difficult and may not be done for years but it is only this kind of painstaking research that will settle the debate once and for all. In the meantime it would be helpful if the medical profession generally were better informed about the evidence that *is* available. There is evidence of various vitamin and mineral deficiencies in many of our western diseases and we need to look at these more closely. The trouble is that like so much biochemical research, the number of variables is enormous and one only ends up treating the 'obvious' deficiencies empirically. There is no reason to believe that because we can readily find a blood deficiency of substance X that giving people more X will cure a given disease. It may well be that substance Y which we don't even know about, let alone can measure, is far more important.

Simple remedies are always appealing, especially for complex problems. Megavitamin therapy is one such simple remedy. Only research will prove whether it is in fact a useful one.

Naturopathy

Definition

A way of treating illnesses which works on the principle that healing depends upon the action of natural healing forces present in the human body.

Background

The concept of *vis medicatrix naturae* – the healing power of nature – is very ancient. It certainly goes back to the time of Hippocrates in 400 BC as Hippocrates himself seems to have been one of the first to realize the importance of nature's own healing powers. To him disease appeared 'not purely as a malady but also, by no means least, as an exertion, an effort of the body to establish the disturbed equilibrium of the function. Recovery is thus shown to be the work of Nature, whose healing powers alone, or supplemented by medical aid, achieve the aim – Nature is the healer of diseases' – according to Dr Max Neuberger, author of *The Doctrine of the Healing Power of Nature through the Course of Time*, 1943.

Paracelsus held that there were two kinds of doctors: 'those who heal miraculously and those who heal through medicine'. Over the centuries that followed, all kinds of theories abounded as to the nature of this healing force. Anton Mesmer (see page 171) called it 'animal magnetism' and Karl von Reichenbach, the celebrated chemist and discoverer of creosote, called it 'odic force' or 'odyle'. Reichenbach made it clear that such a healing force was nothing to do with chemical, electric or magnetic forces as we understand them. Lakhowsky, author of *The Secret of Life*, states that 'the cell-organic unit in all living beings is nothing but an electro-magnetic resonator, capable of emitting and absorbing radiation at a very high frequency.'

Unfortunately, for all our advances in science we are still no nearer knowing the true nature of this healing force, though isolated discoveries are beginning to point the way. One of the most important of these was made by the Russian engineer Semyon Kirlian and his wife Valentina during the 1950s. Using alternating currents of high frequency to 'illuminate' their subjects, they photographed them. They found that if an object was a good conductor (such as a metal) the picture showed only its surface, while the pictures of poor conductors showed the inner structure of the object even if it were optically opaque. They found too that these high frequency pictures could distinguish between dead and living objects. Dead ones had a constant outline whilst living ones were subject to changes. The object's life activity was also visible in highly variable colour patterns.

High frequency photography has now been practised for twenty years in the Soviet Union but only a few people in the West have taken it up seriously. Professor Douglas Dean in New York and Professor Philips at Washington University in St Louis have produced Kirlian photographs and others have been produced in Brazil, Austria and Germany.

Using Kirlian photography it is possible to show an aura around people's fingers, notably around those of healers who are concentrating on healing someone. Normally, blue and white rays emanate from the fingers but, when a subject becomes angry or excited, the aura turns red and spotty. The Soviets are now using Kirlian photography to diagnose diseases which cannot be diagnosed by any other method. They argue that in most illnesses there is a pre-clinical stage during which the person isn't actually ill but is about to be. They claim to be able to foretell a disease by photographing its pre-clinical phase.

But the most exciting phenomenon illustrated by Kirlian photography is the phantom effect. During high frequency photography of a leaf from which a part had been cut, the photograph gave a complete picture of the leaf with the removed part showing up faintly. This is extremely important because it backs up the experiences of psychics who can 'see' the legs of amputees as if they were still there. The important thing about the Kirlian phantoms though is that the electromagnetic pattern can't possibly represent a secondary phenomenon – or the field would vanish when the piece of leaf or leg vanished. The energy grid contained in a living object must therefore be far more significant than the actual object itself.

There are clearly many other bodily phenomena such as this that can and will be explained in terms we can understand but, as with so many similar effects, progress is slow because of scepticism. It seems reasonable to suppose though that there *are* forces in and around living things – forces that we cannot as yet perceive, measure or explain. Some of these forces are probably what naturopaths and others have called the natural healing forces but we're probably centuries away from having any real answers. (For further discussion on this, see page 285.)

What is it?

Naturopathy is a form of medicine practised widely throughout the world although it is often not called by this name outside the West. It is basically concerned with discovering and removing the root cause of disease whether it be chemical (from faulty eating, drinking, breathing or elimination), mechanical (spinal malalignment, muscular tension, stiff joints or bad posture) or psychological. A patient's symptoms help a naturopath to arrive at a diagnosis (which he does to appear medically acceptable rather than because he actually needs to) but don't really concern him much. What he tries to do is to treat the patient and not his symptoms. Naturopaths work on the principle that acute disease is simply a manifestation of the healing forces' efforts to get the body back to normal. Because of this they don't like suppressing symptoms because, they argue, they're there for a reason. 'There's little point giving a man who's bashing his head against a wall a couple of aspirins for his headache,' a leading naturopath explains; 'it's far better to stop him bashing his head. Far too much of modern medicine is involved in giving the aspirin and far too little in finding out why he's bashing his head and stopping him doing it again!' 'The thing is', he continues, 'it's so much easier to dole out drugs than it is to take time to find out what's wrong with a patient's life style. That's a much more tedious job and often the patients won't allow us to do it. Quite frankly, if I were running the whole nation's health along naturopathic lines I would still have to have a pharmaceutical industry even though we don't believe in drugs, simply because the demand for instant, lazy ways out is so enormous.'

How is it done?

A naturopath is really a teacher more than a doctor. Most are not medically trained but do undergo a long and technical training. His training though is aimed at enabling him to assess a patient and then to make suggestions as to what he should do in order to rid himself of his ailments and prevent future ones.

When you go to see a naturopath it's much like going to a doctor but, because a naturopath relies so much more on what the patient tells him, he spends longer taking a history. The patient's story is elicited with greater care and more detail than those with experience of doctors are used to. The naturopath often uses blood tests, X-rays and so on to help arrive at a diagnosis but these are not always necessary. In addition, naturopaths also use osteopathic diagnosis, a method by which they can identify causes of functional and postural derangement which are not diagnosable in other ways. Altered structure and posture are increasingly recognized as being sources of internal body dysfunction, so understandably the naturopath will want to see if there are curable malfunctions that are caused in this way.

Because this combination of naturopathy with osteopathy (see page 231) seems to produce such good results, most naturopaths will assess posture, look for tender areas (especially in the spinal tissues), look for muscular tensions and finally try to seek out any fixed or locked vertebrae. Almost any of these can cause pains in areas of the body not immediately obvious to the layman which can often be helped by correct manipulation of the affected part. In this way naturopaths have a lot in common with teachers of the Alexander Technique (see page 65).

Once the diagnosis is made, the naturopath will take the whole person into account and reorganize his life style – often quite dramatically if he considers it necessary. Diet is about the most important starting point for all naturopaths. They argue that healthy tissues and life's natural healing forces can't work properly if the building blocks – our food – are deficient. No amount of health measures or righteous, healthy thinking can work if the food is inadequate. So food is a starting point in almost every case a naturopath sees. Working on the principle that most of us eat thoroughly unwholesome (and unnatural) foods, the naturopath seeks to re-educate the patient into sensible ways of eating. This doesn't mean they're food freaks or tell you to go out and eat nuts and berries. On the contrary, most naturopaths are very practical – they have to be, because with no medicines to fall back on, they have to get results by persuading people to help themselves, or they're soon out of business. They also advise natural, whole and unrefined foods whenever possible and they encourage the person to take more fresh air, exercise and so on.

Having said this though, some naturopaths also prescribe herbal cures, or use homoeopathic doses of drugs, but these are strictly additions to naturopathy which by definition uses nothing that doesn't come from within the patient. When such remedies are used they are used to mobilize the body's own defences rather than actually to have a positive effect in their own right. Naturopaths are not 'anti-operation' and agree that there are certain conditions for which an operation is necessary. They are convinced though that many conditions requiring operations could have been prevented by healthy living.

As it seems to make little sense to naturopaths to build new health regimes on to a decaying and badly ordered body, they'll often use fasting to clean out the body's metabolic systems first before starting a new approach to diet. By no means all patients that go to naturopaths need to fast and in no way is the fasting like starvation. What they are aiming for is a relative physiological rest for the body so that waste materials can be eliminated before a new diet is begun. Fruit and vegetable juices are taken during such a fast and this alone can produce remarkable results after even only a few days.

Because so many diseases are seen by naturopaths to have originated in the mind, they place great stress on good psychological history taking so that any underlying stresses and traumas responsible for so much disease can be eliminated. Once again the idea is that by freeing the mind from unnecessary tensions the body is freed to heal itself. Any good doctor does this every day and knows just how valuable it can be.

So by all the means at their disposal naturopaths encourage the patient to restore balance and wholeness to his life.

What is it used for?

Naturopathy works particularly well for acute conditions such as sore throats, colitis, gastritis, bronchitis, piles, digestive and liver problems but can also be used for more serious diseases such as tuberculosis. Not all patients with the same disease label get treated the same way for the simple reason that the causes are often so different. 'We're not treating illness,' says a leading naturopath, 'we're inducing health. It's much more positive. Of course we do have our failures like all systems of medicine but at least we haven't done anything positively harmful to the patient. When we do fail it's usually because the patient can't alter his life style along the lines we suggest – after all, it's not easy to give up a stressful job or leave your wife. And this is where doctors can seemingly win hands down because although they don't often make an attempt to change the patient's life they can give him wonder drugs that alleviate the symptoms and everybody – the doctor especially – likes that. In practice he ends up using an endless series of medical crutches because he can't change the circumstances of so many of his patients and simply goes along the path of least resistance. It doesn't solve the patient's problem in many cases though, which simply means he needs more and more crutches in order to cope. We're trying hard to make people more resilient and more self-sufficient.'

Does it work?

Yes it does, as hundreds of thousands of satisfied patients will testify. It is my opinion that naturopathy will go a long way in the relatively near future. People are increasingly disenchanted with drugs and realize that they're better off looking after themselves and preventing disease than trying to get patched up later. It may even be that in the next decade or two as we learn what drugs are really doing to us that there might be a mass move away from drugs for the everyday niggling but inconsequential ailments that take us to our doctors. When this occurs the naturopath will be in even greater demand than he is today.

Negative Ion Therapy

Definition

The use of negatively charged air particles to prevent and cure disease.

Background

Air ions were unknown until the end of the nineteenth century when Elster and Geitel in Germany and Thomson in England independently discovered their existence. Many scientists in the past had proposed that there were electrical forces all around us that had beneficial and harmful effects and perhaps Anton Mesmer was really talking about ions in the air when he was propounding his theories on animal magnetism.

Air molecules are constantly being ionized (i.e. broken down into negatively or positively charged particles) in nature. Energy to do this comes from a variety of natural sources including background radiation, cosmic rays, electromagnetic waves, the sun, lightning and waterfalls. Under certain meteorological conditions both the total number of air ions and the ratio of positive to negative ones change. Most air molecules are not positively or negatively charged; in fact only about 4,000 in every two million, million, million are so charged in pure mountain air but this can rise enormously under unusual natural conditions.

In pure country air, small negative ions (mostly negatively charged oxygen ions) are produced and are present in concentrations of 300–1,000 ions per cubic centimetre of air. This is probably the level at which we were meant to function optimally. As we move into the cities we find that the concentration falls to about half its rural level and that inside air-conditioned buildings there may be a predominance of positive over negative ions because modern air-conditioning units tend to remove small negatively charged ions from the air they purify. An excess of positively charged ions has been shown to cause restlessness, anxiety and depression.

In urban areas small negative ions are constantly being removed from the air by combination with pollutant particles in the atmosphere. A four day study in an industrial area of San Francisco found that as air pollution developed during the working day, the total small ion count fell to less than 80 per cubic centimetre, and that the life expectancy of each ion was reduced as the air became more polluted. All in all then city dwellers get more positive ions and fewer negative ones. This is important because, as we shall see, negative ions tend to have beneficial effects on Man and positive ones harmful effects.

It has been known for years that certain dry, warm winds, peculiar to particular areas of the world, can cause strange mental and physical sensations in those subjected to them. The best example of these is the Sharav in Israel. The most striking features of the Sharav are a sudden rise in temperature, a drop in humidity and an accompanying wind. The interesting thing though is that the Sharav produces illness in 30 per cent of those exposed to it. Although Czermak described this phenomenon over seventy years ago, it wasn't until 1963 that it was discovered that weather-sensitive individuals began to suffer just at the time when the total air ion count began to rise and that they were worst of all when the positively charged ions were at their highest concentration. This occurred twenty-four to forty-eight hours before the weather conditions changed. This phenomenon isn't just found in Israel though. Other examples are the Santa Ana of Southern California, the Chinook of Canada, the Foehn of Switzerland and the Argentine Zonda. From these observations a connection between elevated positive air ion counts and ill health was made.

Professor Sulman, working in Israel, studied people who had

suffered from the Sharav and found that they had remarkably similar signs and symptoms (migraine, nausea, vomiting, swelling, irritability, conjunctivitis, congestion of the respiratory tract and many others). All of these effects can be produced in the body as a response to a naturally occurring chemical messenger called serotonin or 5HT. Sulman then found that not only did his Sharav victims in fact have more 5HT in their urine (in which it is excreted from the body) but also that giving them 5HT antagonists made them better. He also found that he could cure them by giving them air to inhale that was rich in negatively charged ions. So the inescapable conclusion was that this strange wind produced large amounts of positively charged air particles that affected people adversely. These so-called witches' winds around the world have been shown to increase the number of road accidents, violent crimes, suicides and murders and so have led to a very real contemporary interest in 'electricity' in the air.

Historically it was known that certain environments seemed healthier than others. Certain caves, wells, mountains and so on were renowned for their relaxing air and curative properties but until recently no one knew why. Today's modern equipment tells us that it's often the high concentration of negative ions in the air that's doing the good.

Since the original discoveries nearly seventy years ago, the whole subject has until recently had a bad aura, mainly because 'electrical' therapies of the nineteenth century were so plentiful and often so cranky. Electricity was used in party games of this period and numerous quacks produced dramatic and often dangerous demonstrations of the healing power of electricity in an age when electricity was, after all, a relatively new wonder. This led the medical profession to disbelieve anything connected with electrical treatments. The negative ion field suffered a real body blow in the 1950s when unscrupulous businessmen in the USA manufactured so-called ion generators for healing purposes on the back of massive advertising campaigns. The Food and Drug Administration in the USA banned these machines in 1961 because they simply couldn't be proved to have the healing effects claimed and also because they produced harmful ozone as a by-product. This ban which persists until the present day gave the whole subject a bad name.

But as progress was halted in the USA, work continued on negative ion therapy in Russia (which had always been the leader in this field) and in England. Two researchers, C. A. Laws (an electronics engineer) and Dr E. Holiday (a physician), teamed up to produce a new type of ion generator that would be safe and produce no harmful ozone.

There are several methods of producing negative ions instrumentally and they are all basically extensions of the ways they are produced in nature. Ultra-violet light, weak sources of radioactivity, water sprays and high voltage discharges can all be used. The two English workers perfected a high voltage discharge instrument by which large quantities of negatively or positively charged ions could be generated with no danger of producing harmful ozone at the same time. This gave them a distinct lead in the world which has not been surpassed. They then lent thirty trial generators to doctors and other interested groups and sat back expectantly.

They didn't have to wait many months before reports came in of the instrument's effectiveness – in fact they backed up all their hopes which they had based on a survey of the world's existing literature. Here at last was a way of producing a controllable source of negative ions so that they could be applied to prevent and cure disease.

Today there is a mass of scientific and medical research on negative ion therapy from all over the world. The main centres of interest are in the USA, Germany, USSR, Denmark and England. Germany is the only country outside Russia to use ionization therapy on a public scale and there are about thirty electro-aerosol clinics in West Germany. In the USSR, ionization is widely used in hospitals and their medical research on this subject is very advanced compared with ours in the West.

The subject has been boosted somewhat by the work done by NASA in the USA. Their Molecular Biophysics Laboratory has done basic research on the human cell that shows among other things that cancer cells have a greatly reduced electrical charge. This means they clump together instead of being mutually repellent as are normal tissue cells. Dr Kuster at the University of Frankfurt has demonstrated the inhibiting effect of negative ions on the growth of cancerous tumours in mice, so this is obviously an area of great interest for the future. NASA has used negative ionizers to enhance the atmosphere in space craft and has done brain research that shows that performance, work capacity, disposition, reaction times, vitamin metabolism, allergic conditions, pains, burn recovery and healing were all improved in negatively ionized air. Clearly, such a major advance in medical knowledge can't be described as 'cranky' much longer.

How does it work?

Although very considerable research has been done by people such as Professor Krueger in the USA and Professor Sulman in Israel, we are still in the early days of negative ion therapy and a lot more research has to be done. However, there are many actions that negative ions have on the body that can be proven. They definitely do:

1. Reduce heart rate and blood pressure
2. Increase the volume of air breathed at each breath
3. Increase the beating of the tiny cleansing cells that line the respiratory tract
4. Affect the endocrine (hormone-producing) glands
5. Affect the natural rhythms of the brain
6. Reverse the effects produced by positive ions, i.e. the effects of serotonin, as outlined above.

In rabbits, mice and guinea pigs, breathing small negative ions reduces the free 5HT in their body tissues. 5HT levels in the brain have also been shown to be reduced in rats and mice. This is important because we know that 5HT is one of the most important transmitter substances within *our* nervous systems. Because of this apparently beneficial effect of negative ions on transmitter substances in the brain, studies were done to see if human performance could be improved by giving people negative ions. One such study at the University of Guildford in England of forty-five young men in negatively, positively and normally ionized atmospheres proved conclusively that there 'was a highly significant increase in performance of all the tasks in the group exposed to negative ions as compared to the natural environment controls'. These workers also found that there was a significant influence on the normal circadian rhythm of performance. This, they concluded, may mean that negative ions influence the normal circadian rhythm of performance. This is especially interesting because 5HT is known to be involved in controlling circadian rhythms.

Negative ions also produce more alpha activity in the brain and synchronize this activity in the different areas of the brain. Alpha activity is associated with pleasant feelings and a sensation of relaxation so here again is a useful medical application.

So in summary we don't know exactly how it works but we know enough to realize that it's probably mediated via a neurotransmitter substance in the brain which in turn affects the hormones of the body and the nervous system generally. So widespread is 5HT in the body and so important is its role in the lower midbrain (that controls many of our basic bodily functions including sleep and mood) that it seems likely that this is how negative ion therapy works. It may well act locally on cells in other ways too so as to normalize the body's natural healing forces but we're a long way off being able to prove this.

Of course it is possible that it could simply be a placebo effect. After all, about 30 per cent of people react positively to any kind of therapy even if it's useless. Clearly some people react favourably to negative ion therapy on a placebo basis but one scientist (Schulz) claims that 80 per cent of his subjects responded favourably to negative ionization – far too high a proportion to be simply a placebo effect.

Response rates vary but studies have shown that 50–70 per cent of those with respiratory illnesses benefited and 75 per cent of patients with suppurative sinusitis are either 'considerably improved' or 'moderately improved'. Eighty-one per cent of patients with hypertension improved in one study of 200 patients and 40–45 per cent of people with severe headaches get relief. One trial of people suffering from psychoneurosis, fear and apprehension found that 80 per cent showed partial or complete loss of symptoms after therapy.

What is it used for?

Although people report a sense of well-being and relaxation after exposure to negative ions, this is not the sort of indication that is likely to catch the public's imagination. Far more dramatic is its use for asthma, bronchitis, sinusitis, burns, scalds and eczema. With burns and scalds the pain disappears within ten minutes of applying the ions and there is no blistering. Migraine too responds well to this therapy and one particularly stubborn type (Bickerstaff's migrainous neuralgia) responds better to negative ions than to any orthodox medical treatment.

Other conditions that have been shown to be affected favourably by negative ionization are the common cold, some cases of rheumatism, pain, pulmonary tuberculosis and anxiety.

The trouble with any therapy that seems to cure so many things is that the medical profession, which, by and large, thinks of diseases as discrete entities each in its own little pigeon hole, is loath to accept that any 'whole body' treatment could be of value. Certainly, therapies that seem to be 'cure-alls' often turn out to be useless but this can hardly be said to be the case with negative ion therapy. After all, most medicine is empirical. If it works, it works and that's all the patient cares about. It's a mistake to write off a useful therapy because we can't prove *how* it works – if we did this on any scale we'd soon be left with very few of our orthodox medical treatments.

How is it done?

Air ionizers can be used in two ways. The commonest is for the instrument simply to put out ionized particles into the air which is then inhaled. The second way of using them is to direct the output from the instrument directly on to the affected area. This is clearly the method of choice with burns, scalds, eczema, warts and cysts.

Quite simply the patient sits or sleeps in a room fairly close to the ionizer and breathes normally so as to inhale the ions. As small ions are the most active and because they increase in size as they travel away from the generator, best results are obtained with the instrument fairly close to the patient. It's also important that the patient undergoing treatment isn't charged up with static electricity because this prevents the ions from being absorbed by the body. We have all had electric shocks when touching a metal object after walking on a nylon carpet and these are just the sort of electrostatic forces that have to be avoided. This can easily be overcome, though, by giving the patient a small metal electrode to hold. This is connected to an earth point (a radiator or pipe in the home) so ensuring that the negative ions are maximally attracted to the patient's body.

Ion therapy is completely safe as far as we know and there are no side-effects. Respiratory illness responds well to repeated overnight usage – the ionizer is usually placed about four feet from the patient. More concentrated effects can be obtained using a more concentrated beam close to the patient but this sort of treatment should be limited to forty-five minutes at any one session. Two to four treatments can, however, be given in any one day.

The best form of treatment has to be discovered by trial and error in each particular patient. When using an ionizer for general improvement in brain function it should be placed four to six feet away and forgotten.

The benefits can be felt immediately in the case of burns,

some forms of migraine, catarrh and hay fever, but other conditions such as asthma and eczema need longer. Children's colds have repeatedly been cured after one night in ionized airs yet a chronic migraine sufferer may need weeks of treatment before symptoms are lost completely.

Suffice it to say that ionizers really do work. Nearly twenty years of clinical experience of thousands of patients show this to be the case. It's also interesting that the UK manufacturers of the ionizers mentioned earlier get requests from customers to sell back their equipment because they no longer need it. This sort of evidence surprises even the hardiest of negative ion therapists who firmly believed that the effects would be temporary and certainly didn't expect to see long term cures in the medical sense.

What of the future?

Negative ion therapy is now beginning to gain credibility both among doctors and the scientific fraternity. There are moves in the USA to have the ban on ion generators lifted provided this doesn't mean a new generation of machines that produce harmful ozone, and workers in the field see the FDA giving its approval very soon.

There is now so much evidence from all over the world (especially from the UK) that is favourable to negative ion therapy that it must catch on soon. I see a future in the commercial world long before the medical world uses it to anything like its full potential. Employers, keen to alter the environment of their workers, both back to a more natural one and towards one that will have positive effects on their staff, will probably lead the way. The stringent control of air pollutants will also be a hallmark of future industry and this can only lead to a return of air conditions that favour the natural formation of negative ions. Slowly, as urban air approaches that of rural air in its negative ion content, we should see some benefits and a reduction in some of the diseases currently associated with buildings rich in positive ions. Air-conditioning equipment will be modified so as to remove fewer of the small negative ions that are so valuable and undoubtedly the tangible benefits will recommend such new systems to workers and employers alike. Lastly, city authorities and governments will adopt standards for air ionization just as they have for temperature, humidity and air turnover in places where people work. The goal here should be to produce fresh, country-like air for everyone.

Medically, the future is more difficult to foresee. As clinical trials accumulate there will be a move towards the medical applications of negative ion therapy but until the FDA removes its ban no progress is likely in the USA and that is where the new wave of medical applications will come from. The inbuilt conservatism of the majority of the medical profession, even in the UK which currently leads in the technology, will hold back speedy development for several years yet but the beneficial results of this therapy speak for themselves and medical resistance is breaking down far more quickly than to many other alternative medical therapies. Undoubtedly the Russians will continue to lead the field but because of the inaccessibility of their data and the language problems this is unlikely to have much impact on us in the West for some time.

Orgone Therapy

Definition

The use of orgone, usually from an accumulator, to cure certain illnesses.

Background

Dr Wilhelm Reich (1897–1957) was one of Freud's most talented pupils but broke away from him after the publication of his book *The Function of the Orgasm* which, because of its brilliant and outspoken originality, infuriated the puritanical Freud.

Reich wandered from Vienna to Berlin, from Sweden to Norway, and ended up in the USA in 1934 in a place he called Orgonon. Here he set up his own laboratories and research centre into the science of Life Energy. He was undoubtedly a genius but his very weird writings and seemingly bizarre ideas on sex led him to be disregarded by medical and lay people alike. He was ahead of his time though and many of his ideas wouldn't appear so way-out today.

But Reich's main claim to fame was that he believed that he had discovered a new form of fundamental energy which he called Primordial or Cosmic Orgone Energy – orgone for short. Orgone was, he claimed, a continuum of energy that surrounds us all rather like electromagnetic waves do. It is distinct from electromagnetism and penetrates everything to some degree, though at varying speeds. Orgone, unlike kinetic energy, which flows from stronger to weaker parts, flows the other way round. Each substance and living organism has its own capacity for orgone and discharges the surplus. Orgone is always in motion, moves in waves and usually pulsates from east to west. It travels at the speed of light.

Reich said that metal reflects orgone and vegetable matter attracts it and he found that by constructing a box or accumulator made of metal and wood in layers, he could 'concentrate' orgone just like an electrical charge in an accumulator. The orgone so trapped in the accumulator can then be directed via a tube to the outside and used for healing purposes. If a sufficiently large accumulator is built, the patient can be seated inside it. An English doctor, Dr Aubrey T. Westlake, has used such a 'shooter' device to cure pain and promote the rapid healing of wounds and the quick and painless healing of burns and scalds without scarring. A doctor friend of mine with synovitis of the knee was treated by Dr Westlake's orgone 'shooter' and reported that after an initial sensation of coolness, there was definite improvement within half an hour, after which the pain did not return.

During an experiment in 1950 in which Reich was trying to show that orgone could counteract the dangers of radiation, a reaction occurred between orgone and the radium he was using. The Orgone Institute's experimental mice died en masse and many of his workers suffered from radiation sickness. The background radiation count was reported by the *New York Times* to be raised for 600 miles around the Institute and this drew much adverse publicity. Reich had inadvertently created a new substance from the previously harmless (indeed useful) orgone which he called Deadly Orgone (DOR). This was produced by the interaction of orgone and nuclear fission and, he argued, was also being produced by nature in clouds over desert areas the world over. He maintained that because of the increasing numbers of nuclear reactions in the post-war period, orgone in the atmosphere was reacting with nuclear radiation so produced and was collecting as deadly orgone in clouds over deserts. He maintained that DOR was partly responsible for the increase in the area of deserts and their slow but inexorable encroachment on good arable land. While he was working in

Arizona trying to find ways of dispersing these clouds he was arrested for contempt of court.

This arrest came as a finale to a long 'conspiracy' by the authorities to defame and discredit him. In 1947 Reich was the subject of a Federal Food and Drugs Administration investigation but opposition died out in 1950. By 1954 things were on the move again at the FDA and in March an injunction was served on Dr Reich and the Reich Foundation in which 'the defendants were enjoined from distribution of orgone energy accumulators . . . all accumulators to be dissembled, all printed matter regarding these and orgone energy to be destroyed *on the grounds that orgone energy does not exist.*'

As a result of his arrest, all Reich's work was incinerated and as he languished for two years in jail, the Institute was fined very heavily. He died in jail from a heart attack. It has been postulated that he died prematurely (although he was seventy he had described himself as being in extremely vigorous health because of his regular doses of orgone) because of the withdrawal of his regular orgone therapy. Experiments with rats have shown that they can be rendered dependent upon magnetic fields so that if the field is removed they die. Perhaps a parallel phenomenon explains Reich's death.

Does it work?

Except for very small numbers of patients treated by Reich himself (and his records have gone) and those treated by a handful of followers, there is very little evidence on which to assess Reich's orgone therapy. Dr Aubrey Westlake claims he has had excellent results in a restricted group of conditions affecting the skin (mostly burns, scalds and wounds) but clearly a lot more research needs to be done.

Perhaps Reich's theories on cancer therapy deserve further scrutiny if only because his ideas were way ahead of their time and are being borne out to some extent by current discoveries. His theories fit in very well with our understanding that cancer seems to occur in certain emotional states and with the concept that cancer occurs as a result of a breakdown in the body's defences. He wasn't just a theoretician though. He actually did a lot of work with live cell preparations and showed that cancers arose in areas of the body where for some reason orgone was not flowing properly.

This fringe of medicine, like radiesthesia and many others, defies explanation in today's scientific terms. Perhaps one day we will understand. It seems highly likely that Reich was on to something very big indeed when his experiment got out of hand and nearly killed him and all his staff. The incredibly primitive response of the US authorities is scarcely explicable if what Reich was doing was in fact harmless – or if, as they maintained, orgone simply didn't exist. Perhaps this is another example of what many people fear – namely that if a subject looks like producing too many 'waves' in society (e.g. UFOs) then the authorities step in and either ban it or discredit the people working on it. The implications of the discovery of a completely new form of energy such as orgone are enormous – perhaps it was decided that they were too much for us, the public, to handle.

Osteopathy

Definition

A system of medical therapy that employs manipulation of the body and the spine in particular to remedy disease – even when the signs and symptoms seemingly have nothing to do with the spine.

Background

Osteopathy was conceived in the USA by Dr Andrew Still just over a century ago. Still had studied engineering and because of this and his own medical education, he became interested in the human body as a machine. He tried to work out how it was that defective parts would alter the proper functioning of the body in much the same way as they do in a machine with moving parts. His basic theory was that a lot of ailments we suffer from can simply be explained on a mechanical malfunction basis. Still lost all three of his children from meningitis and his disillusionment with orthodox medicine probably dates from this tragedy. His strong Methodist background was his salvation at this time and was also instrumental in his subsequent medical theories.

Still's meticulous research led to his coining the term 'osteopathic lesions'. The word osteopath comes from two Greek words *osteo* (a bone) and *pathos* (disease) but osteopathy isn't strictly to do with diseased bones as such, so the term is misleading. This is especially unfortunate as osteopathy has valid applications for conditions that are seemingly nothing to do with bones as such. An osteopathic lesion is any structural abnormality that leads to functional or organic disease but more of this later.

Theoretically, osteopathy is based on a scientific knowledge of the body and also on zoology and embryology to some extent. Dr Still was a devout Christian though (his father was a clergyman) and he considered the human body to be God's supreme invention and not simply a collection of cells and organs. To Still, therefore, osteopathy also had a mystical and spiritual dimension and he laid great stress on what is called the Total Lesion – a concept which acknowledges that a person may be disturbed biochemically, psychologically and structurally at one and the same time. In order to return the balance of the whole person to normal, the osteopath may have to adjust all these three levels of the body's function. This is called Total Adjustment.

Still's studies and personal endeavours soon paid off. He was quickly able to demonstrate not only that many diseases were related to spinal disorders but that his methods also cured all kinds of non-bony ailments. His insistence that disease is related to the whole body and not simply to a local part of it bears a resemblance to many other branches of fringe medicine and especially to radiesthesia and acupuncture.

His methods were unusual but because he was a doctor, people listened. He demonstrated the 'setting' of bone misplacements to an admiring group of experts and doctors in the State of Missouri.

Even though it was a one-man show early on, slowly others found they too could use his methods and there were soon enough people to form the American School of Osteopathy which still exists today in Kirksville, Missouri.

Osteopathy was first brought to Britain in the early years of this century and in 1917 the British School of Osteopathy was founded.

An osteopath need not be a doctor. Of the 500 or so qualified practitioners in the UK about fifty are medically qualified. The disturbing thing is that only half the lay osteopaths in Britain have had adequate professional training. In the USA there are about 7,000 qualified osteopaths and osteopathy is a very much more accepted part of the medical scene. Most osteopaths in the USA undergo a seven year training which is just as rigorous as and often longer than that of a doctor.

The question of qualifications raises points concerning the degrees and titles one encounters in any branch of fringe medicine and the legal position of osteopaths highlights the position of all non-medical fringe practitioners.

Because doctors are part of a large body of people controlled by ethical and professional organizations and accountable to statutory bodies in the last resort, most of us trust them, quite rightly, although just as with other groups of people there are the bad and incompetent.

Even medically qualified osteopaths do have mishaps and sometimes make mistakes. But when we hear of lay practitioners in fringe medicine harming people we tend to be more readily critical because we feel there is no professional accountability.

An osteopath in the UK practises under common law and is entirely free and independent of any other medical service. He is not a medical auxiliary like a physiotherapist or a chiropodist both of whom have to accept a doctor's diagnosis and act under his instructions.

Many osteopaths would not want to become a part of the National Health Service simply because this would bring them 'under the doctors' and prevent them formulating and acting upon their own opinions. An osteopath receives patients directly, although many doctors send their patients to him on a referral basis. There are parallels here with the chiropractors in the USA (see page 137).

Over the last thirty years there has been a flourishing business in bogus degrees in America and the UK. Thirty-nine American states have banned the practice with some success but it still continues in Britain. The first real outcry came in 1972 when it was found that certain certificates of efficiency as an estate agent had been awarded to a cat.

There were about 200 phoney 'degree mills' in the USA and fifty in Britain at that time, all charging between £5 and £50 for a superbly produced certificate. It has been known for single advertisements for these degrees to bring in as much as $10,000 so it is no surprise that many people have become rich in the process.

The so-called Nebraska College of Physical Medicine at University House, Coventry, sold degrees to people who wanted to be osteopaths or chiropractors. The man who operated this, one of many similar set-ups, was reported in one newspaper as saying, 'I consider this to be a game of harmless bunkology and one that is perfectly legal in this country . . . I get a good deal of satisfaction out of furthering someone's career. My window cleaner asked if I could make him into a brain surgeon. Of course I can't. But I can give him a diploma saying he is so qualified.'

It is just this sort of thing that causes concern about osteopathy.

Someone can set himself up overnight, with or without a purchased degree, and start manipulating people's spines. This is no longer the case in France where osteopathy can be practised only by doctors at special centres. This is the other extreme to the position in the UK where it can be practised by anyone who calls himself an osteopath and sets himself up in a practice. Hopefully, the middle path will prevail in both countries eventually.

But even though some osteopaths and chiropractors (similar to osteopaths but more vigorous in their treatment methods) are unqualified and even potentially harmful, those that are properly trained do an enormous amount of good.

How does it work?

Still studied the anatomy of Man and animals in enormous detail and developed considerable skills in making diagnoses by feeling and touching the body. He could thus judge the speed, quality and heat of the blood pulsating beneath the surface he touched. In 1870 he formulated the 'rule of the artery' which basically stated that 'Whenever the circulation of the blood is normal,

disease cannot develop because our blood is capable of manufacturing all the necessary substances to maintain natural
immunity against disease.'

The theory behind osteopathy is very ancient. The Ancient
Greeks taught that exercise was invaluable for people of all ages.
The Romans put great stress on healthy bodies and Still basically
taught that the body cannot work properly if the fabric is in bad
condition. Much of his writings about the importance of normal
blood flow also seem to indicate that he was thinking of other
body forces flowing in the blood, much like Reichenbach,
Lakhowsky, acupuncturists and others. The recent advent of
'Functional Technique', originating in the USA, very much
underlines this aspect. This type of osteopathy only 'manipulates'
body energy patterns.

To understand how and why much of osteopathy works we
need to bear in mind that Man has only fairly recently (in
evolutionary terms) walked on two feet. Osteopaths argue that
the masses of minor traumas that occur every day of our lives
have very bad effects on our spines which were never meant to
be upright. The discs between our vertebrae, for example, have
become weight bearing – which they never were historically.
Continual strain on these joints makes back pain and sciatica so
common today. Also, they argue, the abdominal organs hang
down abnormally so causing hernias, piles, constipation and
varicose veins.

At a manipulative level osteopathy works by normalizing the
'osteopathic' lesions causing the problem. These lesions can be
of short duration (in which case they are called acute lesions), or
of long duration (chronic ones). A mechanical osteopathic lesion
is simply an area of the body, usually containing a joint, that has
become deranged or involved in strain, thickening of connective
tissues, pain, shortening, swelling or any combination of these
disorders. Should the affected area be close to a nerve root or
artery in the spinal column (as is often the case) then a re-
mobilization of the joint and freeing of the connective tissue can
allow better blood flow not only to local organs but to the nerves

themselves that supply very distant organs. In this way osteopathy can produce dramatic results at great distances from the area under treatment. Osteopathy also works by rebalancing the autonomic (or automatic, background) nervous system that regulates our basic functions like blood pressure, heart rate, breathing and so on. The way that this comes about is described on page 91 under the Alexander Technique, which works in a very similar way.

So, in summary, osteopathy works on several levels, all of which contribute to a normalization of dysfunctioning body parts.

How is it done?

A session with an osteopath starts with a consultation and the taking of a medical history and is usually complemented by physical, laboratory and X-ray diagnosis as the case demands. The osteopath then examines the patient, laying great stress on what he can detect using only his hands. A good osteopath can detect changes in bones, joints, muscles and connective tissues that even experienced doctors can't feel. This is probably the greatest skill that an osteopath has to learn during his training. However good they are with their hands though many osteopaths will still rely on X-rays to some extent.

A treatment session will usually last for twenty to thirty minutes although the patient may need to rest for a while before going back to his daily life. As so many of the mechanical derangements have usually taken years to develop, it's hardly surprising that much osteopathic treatment can take a long time. Several months of the weekly treatments may be necessary but rarely does the treatment go on for years.

Some people wonder if so many treatments are necessary and whether the osteopath is simply asking them to return so that he can keep his appointment book full. This is rather unlikely, especially for a good osteopath, simply because he'll be so pressed by new patients that he's unlikely to hold on to cured ones deliberately.

The treatment consists substantially of manipulation of the affected part or parts of the body so as to relieve the problems and normalize structure and function. Sometimes the corrective forces required are considerable and the patient may feel some pain but usually this is not the case and the treatment is simply at the 'firm pressure' level.

Although Still himself didn't believe that any other therapies were necessary, today's osteopath will be aware of redressing emotional, environmental, dietary and postural balances. Spinal treatment can't work miracles if there are other underlying problems that are at the heart of the patient's disease. In a structural sense, lesions produced by poor posture or continued nervous tension will always recur unless the patient is taught a method of postural re-education such as the Alexander Technique (see page 83). So, like many of his alternative medical colleagues, the osteopath will tend to treat the whole person rather than simply the 'bad back' he came with.

Some patients often go through a period of feeling worse before they feel better. Others get miraculous relief but this doesn't necessarily mean they're cured permanently.

What is it used for?

Every week nearly a quarter of a million people in the UK go to their family doctors complaining of backache.

Because of the inherent weakness of the spine and because most of us in modern society take far too little exercise (which strengthens the spine's supporting muscles) the back is very liable to injury and misalignment even with the slightest provocation. Really fit individuals like athletes don't get a fraction of the back troubles of their more sedentary brothers and sisters because their good muscle tone holds their joints firmly in place.

Most of us with backache go to our family doctors, but because medical schools don't put much emphasis on the recognition and treatment of backache and spinal disorders generally, the average practitioner can often do little to help. So people seek out other sources of relief and turn to osteopaths. It has been estimated that more than a fifth of the population will go to an osteopath at some time during their lives.

Osteopathy uses manipulation to treat a wide range of conditions. Most practitioners spend 60 per cent of their time manipulating the back, but the same treatment to the neck and any other abnormal joint can restore the structure and function of the body to normal. A good osteopath can achieve in minutes what several weeks of bed rest might not resolve.

The scope is even wider though because osteopathy can, in certain cases, help to cure diseases of the internal organs. The nerve supply to the abdominal organs, for example, comes through the spinal cord and manipulation can thus return the nervous pathways, especially the automatic or reflex ones, to normal.

'People often tell me that their indigestion got better after I manipulated their thoracic spine for backache,' says a prominent medical osteopath. 'But I don't use osteopathy to cure diseases like gastric ulcers, although I could, because I think there are better cures at hand.'

Apart from back pain and trouble with other joints, some cases of bronchitis and asthma are alleviated. A relatively new branch of the art is cranial osteopathy in which the bones of the skull are gently manipulated. This is especially helpful for some migraine sufferers who cannot find relief elsewhere, and for certain reversible eye conditions.

The future

Osteopathy is probably one of the fringes of medicine that is closest to and most accepted by the medical profession. More doctors are involved with osteopathy than with any other fringe of medicine and the osteopaths frankly want to keep 'in' with the medical profession. What they do not want is to become part of it – at least in the UK and Australia – because they fear that they'll become second class doctors, whereas today they are independent agents to whom patients come direct.

'The trouble with osteopathy is that, although I believe it works, I cannot prove it scientifically,' says a medical osteopath. 'It is impossible to do good trials because you cannot pretend to be manipulating someone as you can pretend to be giving them a drug when in fact you are giving them a dummy tablet.'

The demands made upon osteopaths, especially the good ones, are so great that they would be most unwilling to give up their busy practices to go into research. There simply are not enough doctors or well qualified lay practitioners to staff the sort of independent research units needed, even if the money could be found, which is unlikely.

Nobody really knows how much of osteopathy works. According to a leading expert in this field, osteopaths in general claim too much for their art.

'There are two really important things to tell people about osteopathy,' the expert insists. 'First, it simply is not proven that osteopathy can cure as much as most osteopaths claim. Second, before going to an osteopath people must go to their doctors so that any treatable disease can be diagnosed and cured. If nothing is found at this screening stage, a well qualified osteopath can be tried.'

Osteopathy isn't in any sense in opposition to orthodox medicine, nor is it incompatible with homoeopathy, acupuncture or many of the other fringes of medicine. In fact many practitioners combine osteopathy with another so-called fringe – naturopathy is a common example. Osteopathy has been helping people for a century and looks set to go on for at least another.

Pattern Therapy

Definition

A family of therapies based on the assumption (often difficult to prove with our present knowledge of science) that patterns or shapes have a critical effect on our lives and can be instrumental in helping cure disease.

Background

The reader will probably find this section one of the most difficult to understand unless he is one of the relatively small number of people who are sensitive to the supersensible forces which surround us. Some people, called 'sensitives', are seemingly more in tune with supernatural forces than others. These people, for example, can see auras around living things; are psychic; experience telepathy; can easily be trained to develop their psychic skills; can learn to feel colours; are sensitive to supernatural phenomena not usually perceived by the rest of us; or are natural healers. Some fortunate people combine many of these skills whilst others seem to have developed one in particular. It is highly likely that we are all capable of an enormous range of psychic abilities and perceptions but that in most of us they simply aren't developed. Many people working in this field feel sure that over the next century or two, man will emerge from his current developmental phase in which the intellect is the dominant factor and progress to the next phase in which his perception of spiritual and supersensory phenomena will be developed. I for one hope they are right because we are certainly finding very few real answers with our current reductionist approach to medicine and a greater understanding of supersensible forces would be a great help. The patching up we do (both physically and biochemically with surgery and drugs respectively) seems extremely naive and time wasting when we compare it with the more basic considerations contained in ancient medical texts. Much of what was written thousands of years ago in ancient Chinese, Tibetan, Indian and Japanese medicine still stands today but the great dimension they had and which we have lost is the spiritual one.

Back to patterns though. The ancients realized the power of certain shapes and patterns both over their spiritual lives and in the realm of healing. The ancient Egyptians and subsequently the Greeks understood the importance of patterns or shapes – hence their beautiful buildings which were deliberately constructed to carefully calculated dimensions. About fifty years ago, a Frenchman, M. Bovis, noted that small animals which had died in the Great Pyramid of Egypt had not decayed but had, in spite of the considerable humidity, mummified. A Czech engineer connected this observation with his finding that razor blades remained sharp for longer if they were kept under a pyramidal cardboard object aligned to magnetic north. (For more details of this, see Pyramid Healing, page 253.) This led to considerable speculation and research into the significance of the pyramid as a shape. Certain shapes, and pyramids in particular, it seems, have the power to concentrate particular wavelengths of the earth's electromagnetic and other waves to produce extraordinary effects. How this happens is not known but it is a fact nonetheless.

There is considerable research into the importance of shape and form and any good designer will be able to predict the reception of specifically shaped objects by his public. An interesting study of over 1,000 people carried out by one of the world's leading colour therapists, Theo Gimbel, found that out of nine shapes (varying from a straight line, through a circle, a curved and wiggly line, to a pentagram) the pentagram was the favourite of over a third of the subjects.

It has been known for centuries that the shape of buildings affects their occupants. The pyramids of Egypt, the Middle Eastern mosques, the Taj Mahal and certain cathedrals in France are all examples of such buildings. People (especially the sensitives I have described) are often aware of the effect of the form of a building upon them – indeed many of us when looking over a potential new home get bad or good 'vibrations' about it. The proportions of many famous buildings have been copied by succeeding generations and much of their success appears to centre around the fact that they are based on the golden mean ratio 1 to 1.618. This ratio has been used to produce a series of harmonious spatial relationships for thousands of years. Le Corbusier, the distinguished French architect, embodied some of this thinking in his work too and many contemporary artists, architects and designers use the golden mean ratio in their work, often quite intuitively.

But it's not just buildings whose shapes influence their contents. A French yoghurt manufacturer patented a special container because its shape increased the bacterial action that made the yoghurt; mice with identical wounds heal faster if they are living in spherical cages; schizophrenic patients improve if they live in trapezoidally shaped wards; and the taste of beer is altered if it is stored in rectangular rather than rounded barrels.

The pattern or shape of a thing may be far more important than we at present realize, but there's no point in confining our horizons to shapes that are big enough to see. If visible objects have properties that depend to some extent on their shape, so might invisible or microscopic matter, according to experts in this field. After all, even sub-atomic particles in every substance of the physical world conform to recognizable patterns (of energy rather than solid form in this case). In fact, once we start to analyse anything deeply enough it can be reduced to molecules and then to atoms and finally to sub-atomic particles . . . all of which exist not in a random form but in very strict patterns or shapes.

Much alternative medicine may in fact work because of

patterning. Dr A. T. Westlake, an English physician living in Hampshire, is arguably the world's leading expert in the importance of patterns. During the 1950s he and a small research team devised and tested certain patterns and found them useful as aids to psionic medicine (see page 246). Westlake found that having chosen the appropriate Bach (see page 118) or homoeopathic (see page 175) remedy, with the patient's sample placed at the centre of a particular three-dimensional pattern or model for a radiesthetically predetermined time, he could transmit the remedy to the patient. He claims that certain patterns need actual remedies to be placed on them, whereas other more complex dynamic ones need only the written name of the remedy to be placed in the right position on them. In order to understand this better, the reader should turn to the section on radionics (page 276). Westlake and his colleagues claim 300 successful cures using these patterns which incidentally were revealed in dreams to one of the team over a twelve month period. Nobody has since taken them up and used them except Malcolm Rae, a British radionic researcher who has extended the concept of patterns by developing a method whereby the archetypal pattern of many homoeopathic remedies can be ascertained and, if magnetically energized, imprinted on water or inert lactose tablets for administration to patients directly or radionically. This method of preparing homoeopathic remedies has been thoroughly tested over a decade and is now widely used.

The old Doctrine of Signatures (see page 165) is also closely linked with patterns but it's probably fair to say that those who proposed the Doctrine were not thinking along the same lines as we are today. Theirs was a much more simple idea – that a plant or part of a plant that looked like a human organ would have effects on that organ. To a certain extent this principle still applies today with placebo activity in which an inactive tablet, looking like a drug, has the effects of a drug.

Westlake sees pattern as a force in its own right and uses it to explain for example how radionic instruments work (see page 281). As a radionic instrument contains no electrical or electronic circuitry and certainly no means whatsoever of actually broadcasting anything in terms we would understand, Westlake argues that it works simply because of the patterns selected on the dials. These patterns then take upon themselves a power to energize or potentize a remedy (which can then be given to the patient as a tablet) or to transmit the treatment to the patient directly along wavelengths that we don't yet understand. The trouble with all of this is that the pattern of thought itself enters into the treatment. In fact, he argues, it could be that all kinds of healing are carried out by positive healing thought transfer. This seems very strange to most of us who are unaware of the relationships between our mental states and spiritual conditions, but I go into much more detail on page 277). Any placebo study (in which people with real symptoms are given dummy tablets) proves that the healing power of the doctor has somehow been transferred to the patient, as a large proportion of the patients get better on these inactive tablets. We're coming to realize, albeit very slowly, that the power to heal, by whatever means, might well be closely allied to thought transfer. The healer (who may or may not be a doctor) wishes his patient well, transfers a healing pattern to the tablet (which is either active or inactive) and, if the patient's body is in a condition to receive the therapy, its own individual healing force – the *vis medicatrix naturae* (life's intrinsic healing force, see page 211) – gets to work. This doesn't of course mean that an aspirin tablet has no pharmacological effects but simply that it acts in the human body to produce both these effects and a normalization through the body's own healing powers.

In parallel with this a patient given a placebo himself believes the placebo is doing him good and so imparts considerable value to it in his own mind. This concentration of healing thought on the placebo may well potentize it (in much the same way that homoeopathic remedies are potentized) and so make it a useful agent.

Even some of the so-called potent drugs of today may act along these lines. Remember even before the days of antibiotics people didn't automatically die of severe infections – doctors and other healers could often stimulate the body's own resources to heal itself.

Although we don't as yet know much about it, it seems highly likely to me that patterns will be found to be more important than we have ever imagined. Homoeopathic potentization, in which great dilutions of substances become, under the right conditions, highly potent in the body, can also be explained by patterning. Just as with the Bach remedies (see page 118), a homoeopathic remedy imparts its intrinsic energy pattern to the patient and I like to think of the information transferred (as patterns of energy) as a signpost. These energy patterns have no direct effect in themselves but rather signpost the body's natural healing forces to get going on the curative process. It is possible that all remedies work this way and may help explain why it is that one can cure a given symptom (for instance, a headache) by acupuncture, Shiatsu, aspirin, homoeopathy or a host of other ways. Clearly, in such a case, they all produce the same end point but no one has ever suggested that they might all actually work *in the same way* – that is, by acting as energy pattern signposts to the body to set itself right again. The fact that certain biochemical values in, for example, the brain are abnormal in specific 'pathological' conditions may well not be the *cause* of the disease as we know it, but may be the *result* of the disease and that's why they return to normal when a drug or other treatment is given.

Today, we're still scratching at the surface of all this. There must be a link between all the healing arts and sciences. Perhaps patterning is that link.

Psionic Medicine

Definition

A system of medicine substantially devised by an English surgeon, Dr George Laurence, that uses the best of orthodox medicine in conjunction with the radiesthetic faculty in an attempt to get at the fundamental cause of disease.

Background

George Laurence qualified in medicine in London in 1904 and went on to hold several hospital appointments and to build up a brisk private practice. He was left to carry on a general practice in Wiltshire at the start of the First World War during which time he also held consultative appointments locally. It was during his forty years in general practice that he first developed the concept of psionic medicine but it wasn't until he retired in 1954 that he could devote himself to it full time. Other interested doctors joined him in 1968 to form the Psionic Medical Society which is still gaining strength. Having said this though, there are fewer than twenty doctors practising psionic medicine in the UK today and probably only a handful elsewhere throughout the world.

Psionic medicine (so called because the Greek letter psi has been widely used in the context of psychic and paranormal phenomena) is not simply an extension of orthodox medicine, nor is it a kind of super radiesthesia (see page 261) but is an integrated system linking homoeopathy, radiesthesia and orthodox medicine. It is based on a careful and well researched application of paranormal faculties and involves a long training after obtaining a medical degree. Laurence maintained that psionic medicine had to be practised by trained doctors because they have a grounding in basic anatomy, physiology and bio-chemistry and are thus able to ask the right questions in order that psionic medicine can supply the answers.

We saw in the Introduction that much of our disease burden can't readily be explained by the reductionist approach of western medicine and that we need to accept the existence of a higher level of intuition or 'etheric force'. Psionic medicine accepts all this as basic and grafts on other, more radical ideas. One of the most revolutionary of these is the theory of miasms.

The concept of miasms was the creation of Hahnemann, the founder of homoeopathy. Although he had worked out the basis of homoeopathy by 1810 in his *Organon der rationelle Heilkunde* which was published when he was fifty-five, it wasn't until much later in his long and eventful life that he elucidated the theory of miasms. Over the years he had found that although his homoeo-pathic remedies produced excellent results in acute conditions, many chronic conditions were affected temporarily and then reappeared. He reasoned that these recurring troubles were caused by a kind of unknown 'primitive malady' that disrupted the body's natural curative forces so that they were unable to restore the body to health as they normally would. This idea was scarcely new as Thomas Sydenham, the father of British medi-cine, had proposed 200 years earlier that illness is itself a kind of cure – an attempt by the body to get the vital healing forces back to normal. Hahnemann developed his ideas and suggested that there were things called miasms that so deranged the body's vital energy forces that the body not only failed to recover from certain diseases but also became more susceptible to other seemingly unrelated conditions.

As I explained in the Introduction, it is helpful to think of the body as two closely interlinked and interdependent systems – the physical body and the etheric or supersensible body. The physical body behaves in accordance with the laws of nature, cause and effect and so on. The treatment for disorders of the body has traditionally been to produce another effect with some sort of medical therapy. But with the etheric body, things are rather different. To quote from *Psionic Medicine* by J. H. Reyner, written in collaboration with its founder Dr George Laurence, 'It is evident that the material structure can be affected by influences of a superior order, while still being subject to the laws of physical cause and effect, and any derangement of this underlying energy pattern will create effects in the material body which cannot be interpreted or treated, in terms of physical cause.'

It is these derangements that are Hahnemann's miasms, according to psionic doctors. These lingering distortions of the body's etheric forces are of course unrecognizable by orthodox medicine yet can be detected by supersensible methods such as radiesthesia.

To be more specific, an infection such as tuberculosis disturbs the vital energy forces of the body in such a way as to affect the etheric body too. Over a period of time and with good orthodox treatment the physical body becomes overtly 'well' but the etheric body carries the 'memory' of the old TB. This weakening of the system then causes illnesses, not necessarily in the person himself but even in his successors (because the etheric body is timeless).

According to Laurence and other key workers in this field, the two main hereditary miasms are those of syphilis and TB. The acquired ones come mostly from the acute infections of childhood such as measles, whooping cough and chicken pox. Dr Aubrey Westlake, a founder member of the Psionic Medical Society, told me how enormously widespread the TB miasm is, for example. 'There is a number of common diseases today that are in fact manifestations of the hereditary TB miasm,' he said. 'The list includes asthma, eczema, hay fever, other allergies, pharyngeal and sinus trouble, migraine and mental illness of various kinds. There is also a link between leukaemia, Hodgkin's disease, diabetes, varicose veins, arterial disease and the TB miasm. A very important effect of the TB miasm though is that it makes the patient more likely to retain toxic substances produced by common infections. This is especially true of the acquired miasms of measles.' He then went on to say how measles is now known to affect the brain and to cause abnormalities on the electroencephalogram but that this came as no surprise to psionic doctors who had often seen this link psionically before orthodox medicine caught on to it.

Although most orthodox doctors would shrink at the word miasm, they are probably slowly beginning to catch on to the whole subject but in other terms. In 1969 US government scientists reported a breakthrough in virus research which began to shed light on a variety of illnesses from multiple sclerosis to some forms of cancer and Parkinson's disease. The report suggested that a host of still unsolved maladies might be due to 'smouldering' viruses left over from an infection very early in life . . . such as measles. Scientists at the National Institute for Health found, after four years of research, that the virus responsible for a rare kind of brain disease causing the deaths of 100–200 young Americans each year was identical with the virus long known to cause measles. In 1974 an article in *Scientific American* drew attention to 'certain viruses that persist in their host without giving rise to the usual signs of infection. Evidence is accumulating that such viruses can cause or trigger degenerative disease in man.' The article goes on to show that preliminary evidence suggests that 'slow' viruses (which probably are as close to Hahnemann's miasms as we are likely to get) might be important in diseases such as diabetes, rheumatoid arthritis, leukaemia and multiple sclerosis.

But etheric imbalances don't only occur as a result of infections and diseases as we recognize them. Psionic doctors put great emphasis on, for example, aluminium poisoning. Aluminium, it appears, emits 'radiations' which are not tolerated at all well by the human body. Although the blood levels of aluminium of people who eat out of aluminium cookware may be normal (and hence raise no suspicion in the minds of orthodox medics) these people respond dramatically to the removal of aluminium from their diets. This is a kind of reverse homoeopathy – in other words a tiny amount of highly potent aluminium is having an effect on the person's etheric body and can, according to Dr H. Tomlinson in his book *The Divination of Disease*, produce duodenal and gastric ulcers, liver and gall-bladder problems, rectal diseases and cancer. But it's not only aluminium that can be so troublesome according to these doctors; lead too can have a similar disruptive effect on the etheric body.

The last main foundation stone of psionic medicine is an embodiment of McDonagh's Unitary Theory of Disease. J. E. R. McDonagh, a surgeon like Laurence, proposed that all disease could be linked to basic disruptions in the body's vital energy forces. These disruptions did one main thing, he maintained – they distorted protein production in the body. And since protein production is at the very heart of our 'structure', this is what disease is really all about. He saw all disease as varying degrees of protein imbalance – cancer being the most extreme imbalance of all.

Although this sounds ridiculous to many doctors and scientists, it is far more sensible than it at first seems and is being backed up by modern molecular chemical research. McDonagh argued that as the physical world is so transitory (our bodies are after all made up of chemicals which in turn consist of ever-changing submicroscopic electrons) there must be a baseline primitive activity (the etheric force field) from which all matter and energy are produced. He then postulated four increasing orders of physical cycles. The first creates sub-atomic particles of extremely short lifespan (an electron probably 'lasts' for 1/10,000th of a second) which are constantly being replenished. The second cycle builds these into three distinct groups of atoms that he calls radiation, attraction and storage. The third cycle makes simple molecules and the fourth creates basic protein building blocks for living matter. The fifth and sixth cycles organize all this protein into useful body organs and other structures.

McDonagh's thesis then was that all disease comes about because the protein in the blood (which will eventually be used to reform broken down tissue) has lost its powers to 'attract nourishment', store energy or radiate it to the tissues.

This theoretical base plus a considerable skill with a pendulum is what the psionic practitioner has to learn – it's no wonder there are so few of them.

How is it done?

The practice of psionic medicine depends upon a good knowledge of orthodox medicine and an intuitive ability to be able to examine witnesses and prescribe remedies radiesthetically. The basic methods are very much like the best of radiesthesia. The doctor, using a pendulum as an indicator, asks it a series of mental questions using a witness from the patient or the patient himself and lets the pendulum tell him the answer (see page 268 for more details of the use of the pendulum). Although the psionic doctor's medical background enables him to ask the right questions, he doesn't necessarily get the answers he'd expect, simply because he's tapping another dimension of information – the supersensible forces and not a memory bank in his head or in a library.

Colour plays an important part in psionic diagnosis. Laurence found that infections reacted very specifically to different colours and soon he developed a classification of disease according to these colours. This helped him take a short cut to a diagnosis since he was able to tell from the reaction of the patient's witness to a given colour which broad group of diseases he was most likely to be suffering from. This simply cut down the otherwise large number of witnesses that would have had to be tested to link one to the patient's disease.

Psionic medicine puts great importance on actually arriving at a diagnosis properly obtained by a detailed 'normal' medical history and subsequent radiesthetic techniques. Its practitioners put great stress on inherited and acquired miasms as we have seen and will often try to eliminate these basic faults before embarking on any treatment aimed at the secondary manifestations of these

miasms. But psionic medicine also comes into its own when deciding upon treatment. Prescribing the right homoeopathic remedy is
often haphazard but by using radiesthetic techniques the exact
remedy can usually be arrived at without recourse to trial and
error. Laurence and his followers have built up an enormous
experience with psionic medicine and claim to be able to diagnose
and treat most conditions, be they acute or chronic.

Psionic doctors may have to treat several conditions in any
one patient but each is tackled systematically in order of its
importance. Care has to be taken to watch the patient in the
early days of the treatment because homoeopathic aggravation
can occur. This is a well recognized worsening of the patient's
condition as detoxification takes place and is a part of the life
forces being normalized but can cause concern to the patient if
he hasn't been prepared for it.

What is it used for?

Perhaps the main advantage of psionic medicine is its ability to
treat chronic states, normally thought of as incurable by orthodox
medicine, by ascertaining the basic causal factor involved. As so
many diseases are caused, according to this school of medicine,
by inherited miasms undetectable by doctors using orthodox
methods, a simple normalization of the harmonies of the body's
energy patterns (etheric forces) will cure a large percentage.
This is almost always achieved using radiesthetically prescribed
homoeopathic remedies.

There is no standard procedure as such in psionic medicine as
by definition each patient is treated as a unique individual. This
means that treatments are unique too although there will clearly
be overlap in very similar clinical cases.

Psionically treated patients are numerous now and conditions
as chronic as asthma, eczema, brucellosis, depression, migraine,
aluminium sensitivity, skin conditions, schizophrenia, Hodgkin's
disease, physical and mental retardation, coeliac disease, general
debility and dental caries have been treated or prevented.

Pyramid Healing

Definition

A potential healing method using pyramidal structures.

Background

The exact significance of the pyramids of Egypt has baffled scientists and archaeologists for centuries. What we do know is that the Great Pyramid at Giza is *not* simply a super tomb for a great Pharaoh – it is much more. For a start, it is by far the biggest building ever constructed by Man. Although it was a tremendous height when constructed, it has been surpassed many times since in the modern world (it is only as high as a forty-eight storey office block), but its base covers an area of 14 acres. It is 450 feet high and contains 90 million cubic feet of stone. This is hard to visualize in isolation but would build thirty Empire State Buildings; a wall three feet high and one foot thick, 5,300 miles long; or all the cathedrals, churches and chapels in England built since the time of Christ. It contains an estimated 2,400,000 stones, ranging in weight from 2½ to 70 tons each.

The Great Pyramid is the finest of the original eighty or so that were built in Egypt, thirty of which still stand today. Apart from its size it is remarkable in many other ways. For a start, the construction of such an enormous building two thousand years ago almost defies imagination. We still don't know how such an edifice was built, taking, as it must have done, many years, hundreds of thousands of men, millions of logs (for rollers to move the stones) and an enormous navy of barges and other transport to bring the stone from as far as 500 miles away. The more we discover about the Great Pyramid, the more baffling it all seems. Who could have organized such a project; how were the people fed, considering the whole project took place in a vast desert; where did they get the timber; how did they place 70-ton stones so accurately; how did they joint them so finely that a piece of baking foil can't be inserted between the stones? The questions keep on coming. Eric von Daniken has written books (such as *Chariot of the Gods*) suggesting that this was too great a feat for humans alone and that they must have had help from outer space.

Be this as it may, there are more uncanny facts yet to come. For a start, the Great Pyramid is aligned so exactly to magnetic north that it defied modern measuring systems. Until very recently it was thought that the pyramid was slightly off this true north–south axis but with the development of more sophisticated measuring methods, it was realized that the Ancient Egyptians had got it right and that we had been wrong all these years! The pyramid is constructed with very special dimensions and proportions. Professor Jacob Bronowski, the late author and TV personality, said in his book *The Ascent of Man* that the Egyptians were the first to discover geometric symmetry – the scale of proportions that rules the 'harmony of nature'. So basic are the 3–4–5 unit relationships found in the pyramids that scientists engraved the same triangular figures on a plaque sent into space on a space rocket as a means of communication with life on other planets. Nothing about the Great Pyramid is accidental. Its position is the exact centre of the earth's land mass. The north–south axis, which is 31°9′ east of Greenwich is the longest land meridian and the east–west axis, 29° 58′ 51″ north, is the longest land parallel. The weight of the Great Pyramid is exactly one thousand trillionth of the weight of the earth, and enables us to calculate the distance of the earth from the sun. Using the pyramid, the figure for this distance comes to 93 million miles and using our latest space probes it comes to 92,900,000 miles.

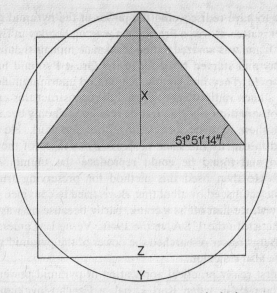

*The essential measurements of the Great Pyramid which must
be reproduced in any healing pyramid*

The astronomical position of the pyramid is also no accident,
and the design seems to have been about 4,200 years ahead of its
time in this respect. But it's in its proportions that it seems to be
so extraordinary. There are any number of ways of constructing
a pyramidal structure – the base and height are infinitely
variable. The Great Pyramid though is of very special dimensions. The height (X) of the pyramid is the radius of a circle
whose circumference (Y) is the same as the circumference of
the square base (Z) of the pyramid. Lines drawn from the axis
to the centre of the vertical sides of the square (see diagram)
form an angle of 51° 51′ 14″. These proportions are what makes
the Great Pyramid, unique in its time, so important today. 'But
what on earth has all this to do with medicine?' I can hear you
saying.

The story goes back to the early 1930s when Antoine Bovis

claimed to have rediscovered the power of the pyramid's shape to affect matter. Bovis, a Frenchman, was on holiday in Egypt in the 1930s and was amazed to find that small animals that had lost their way and starved to death in the Great Pyramid had not decomposed. They had simply dehydrated and mummified. As he was a keen radiesthetist he tried to reconstruct this extraordinary observation when he returned to Paris, if only because he felt sure there must be some strange forces at work. He built a pyramid to exactly the same proportions as those of the Great Pyramid and found he could reproduce the mummification process. He then used this method for preserving fruit and vegetables. Amazed by all of this, Bovis tried to convince people but they wrote him off as a crank, partly because he was also a radiesthetist. In the USA, in the 1940s, Verne L. Cameron and Ralph Bergstresser researched the power of the pyramid's shape but were also ridiculed.

The first really practical application of pyramid power came in the late 1940s when Karl Drbal, a Czechoslovakian radio technician, patented a cardboard pyramid-shaped razor blade sharpener. This is especially remarkable because in Czechoslovakia they don't give a patent until the invention has been tried and proved to be of value. One of the distinguished scientists on the patent board used the razor blade sharpener with astounding results. After that it took ten years of research by top metallurgists to find out how it worked. These distinguished metallurgists found that water can reduce the strength of steel by up to 22 per cent. They found that worn razor blades had minute pockets of moisture in the edge which served to further blunt the razor. On placing the razor under the pyramid structure being tested (with both razor and pyramid aligned due north–south), these pockets of microscopic water were dried out and the razor retained its sharpness. They postulated that there was some kind of force field produced in the pyramid itself that could cause this electromagnetic dehydration. The Pharaoh's razor blade sharpener is now widely available and prolongs the life of a normal blade for anything up to four months if the experience of a friend of mine is anything to go by!

So this and other remarkable findings led people to look at why this might be happening. Two pyramidologists, Bill Kerrell and Kathy Goggin, have conducted numerous experiments in the USA with remarkable results. They find they can alter the taste of food (for the better) by placing it under a pyramidal structure. This makes coffee less bitter; improves the taste of wine; lowers the acidity of fruit juices; improves the taste of frozen foods and a host of other things. Their book *The Guide to Pyramid Power* tells in great detail how these things can be achieved and also outlines their experiments (now replicated with great success by distinguished experts) on enhancing plant growth under pyramids.

But not only can plants and organic matter be influenced by pyramid-shaped structures – so can we human beings.

What is it used for?

Sophisticated biofeedback equipment shows that a trained meditator (or anyone who has been trained to control his brain wave patterns) is influenced by the lowering of an open structured pyramid over his head. Experiments carried out by Kerrell and Goggin used experienced meditators who were wired up to an electroencephalograph machine, which measures the patterns of waves produced by the brain. The subjects were blindfolded and the base line of the brain waves recorded. Then, unknown to them, a pyramid was lowered over them. After about thirty to forty-five seconds, the alpha and theta waves in the brain increased in frequency and were more than double the normal amplitude. Sometimes the alpha activity (the brainwave so sought after by biofeedback experts, see page 128) was so great that it shot off the top of the recording scale. But not only were there remarkable changes on the EEG – the subjects themselves noticed subjective differences when they were under the pyramid. Most frequently reported sensations were a sense of weightlessness, tingling, warmth, tranquillity and relaxation, dreams, graphic visions and time distortion. A few subjects experienced even more extraordinary phenomena including clairvoyant and clairaudient experiences.

Other experiments have shown that people sleeping with a pyramid over their heads need fewer hours sleep and that they awake considerably more refreshed.

Kerrell and Goggin have carried out pyramid tests with children who, they reasoned, would be far more reliable witnesses than adults who are conditioned to reject or at least be sceptical of new phenomena. They took children (who knew nothing about pyramids, fairly obviously) and on a very casual basis gave them the opportunity of going in or out of one placed on the ground in their own back gardens. When the children were inside they were asked very casually if they'd like to stay in there and what if anything it felt like. Only five of the eighteen children tested noticed no change at all. Many felt 'warm all over', body tingling and other sensations. One hyperactive child in particular was very much happier under the pyramid and was able to stay calm and read school books for longer than ever before.

Water that has been placed under a pyramid loses its chlorine taste and, if one experiment is to be believed, might actually have curative properties. A nine-year-old girl had a number of mosquito bites. The experimenters rubbed one of the bites with tap water and another with pyramid water. The girl immediately reported that the pyramid water had stopped the itching. The experiment was then repeated with the girl unable to see which water was being used and she still obtained repeated relief from the pyramid water and no effect from ordinary tap water. Clearly this needs repeating and further research is essential before any real claims of a medical application for pyramid water can be made.

Some researchers claim that pyramids put a brake on the ageing process and certainly some lowly forms of life have been positively affected by pyramids. However in spite of the astounding finding that the skin cells from a 3,000-year-old Egyptian mummy were still capable of life, any claims that pyramids prolong human life must by treated cautiously until much more research is done. Anecdotal reports suggest that women who have been sleeping under a pyramid for four to sixteen weeks notice that their menstrual periods are altered. Many said they were free from pains and cramps and the duration of bleeding was also reduced in several of them.

How does it work?

Nobody knows as yet for sure how it works but it seems likely that certain electromagnetic waves are concentrated and condensed by the particular configuration of a pyramid. Conventional magnetism may be involved in the pyramid's working too because a Gauss meter, placed at the centre of even a non-magnetizable pyramid (one made out of card for instance), shows a positive reading which increases in strength as the pyramid is brought into north–south alignment. Greater readings were produced with metal pyramids but even this is strange because classical magnetic theory would have it that the magnetic materials of the frame should shield the interior of the pyramid from magnetic forces. The pyramid shape itself then seems to attract more than normal of the earth's magnetic forces. But magnetism isn't the only explanation of pyramid power because exactly similar magnetic fields don't produce the same effects as those produced under a pyramid. This seems to confirm that pyramids accumulate several different types of energies. It may be that the benefits derived from pyramids have something to do with the balance of negative and positive ions in the air (see page 217) as pyramids seem to produce some of the beneficial effects found with negative ion therapy.

It'll probably be decades before pyramid power is really understood but there certainly seems to be enough evidence to make further study well worthwhile. It's quite likely that advances in the near future will come from industry rather than medicine. In the USA, plant growers have already reported increases of 150 per cent in growth rates under pyramids and there are also pyramid-shaped schools, warehouses and recreation areas in existence. Unfortunately as with so many exciting 'new' discoveries, rogues and unscrupulous businessmen latch on and give the subject a bad name. People claim to have machines to measure pyramid energy though in fact this can't yet be done. It is possible that some instrumentation exists in the USSR but only because they've been working on the problem for years. The Soviets have extensive research going on into pyramid energies at a large pyramid research department at Leningrad University. Many new pyramid-shaped products are constantly being launched in the USSR.

Claims such as 'It makes your hair grow faster and thicker'; 'It increases crop yields by three times'; 'The pyramid will correct faulty vision and damaged hearing'; 'Will make you more intelligent'; 'Will increase your sex drive' have all been made but without foundation.

I feel we're on the brink of some exciting discoveries about pyramid power in medicine but only time and the work of a few far-sighted doctors will tell.

Radiesthesia

Definition

The use of dowsing (an old Cornish word meaning striking) or divining to diagnose disease and select remedies. (See also Psionic Medicine and Radionics.)

Background

Dowsing is a very ancient pastime. Neolithic man probably knew about its uses and the Ancient Egyptians definitely did. In spite of this though there was no mention of dowsing in European literature until 1240 and the first English language reference to the subject was in 1638 in a book written in Latin by Robert Fludd. In 1639 Gabriel Platts wrote of 'A Discovery of Subterraneall Treasure. The operation with the Virgula Divina is thus to be performed – I cut a rod of Hassel, I tied it to my staff in the middle with a strong thread so that it did hang even, and carried it up and downe the mountaines and it guided me to a veine of lead ore.' Dowsing was at this time considered magical – a manifestation of God, the Devil or other spirits.

But although individuals like Platts were dowsing using hazel twigs, it didn't really catch on until the nineteenth century when studies on the continent of Europe and in England began to show its great potential. In 1897 Professor William Barret F.R.S. published a paper in the *Proceedings of the Society for Psychical Research* entitled 'On the so-called Divining rod or Virgula Divina – a scientific and historical research as to the existence and practical value of a peculiar human faculty, unrecognized by science, locally known as dowsing, with letters from 208 correspondents describing 140 cases of water finding by the 46 professionals and 38 amateur dowsers in 256 localities'. At this time the only possible use for dowsing seemed to be for the location of underground water or mineral ores but this paper and another by the same author in 1900 put dowsing on the scientific map. These papers were eventually combined into one book in 1926 – *The Divining Rod*.

Before we go on any further with the story of medical dowsing it might be helpful to describe how people dowse for something relatively simple like water. The hazel twig, branch, or other divining apparatus (if it is forked or has two limbs) is held in both hands as the person who is dowsing walks over the area suspected of having the stream or mineral deposits beneath. As he approaches the dowsable substance the rod moves, vibrates or oscillates of its own volition and so leads the dowser to his quarry. On rare occasions the movement of the rod may be so vigorous that it flies clean out of the dowser's hands. Metal rods, coathangers, walking sticks and pendulums have been used instead of twigs of wood – every dowser claiming particular benefits for each type of divining instrument when dowsing for different things.

But back to the development of dowsing. Although early this century dowsing was beginning to acquire some scientific credence it was still regarded by most people as a sort of funny game or party trick rather than as a serious or useful procedure. In 1933 the British Society of Dowsers was formed 'to encourage the study of all matters connected with the perception of radiation by the human organism with or without instruments'. The early members of the Society were only interested in developing dowsing for its classical use – i.e. the locating of water and mineral ores – but soon a controversy blew up as to how it worked and like most controversies it was the starting point for far greater advances than those involved at the time realized. The great question of the day was whether dowsing was a physical phenomenon explicable in terms of electromagnetism or was mainly a psychic phenomenon. Much of the confusion was cleared up in a book written in 1949 by Maby, *The Physics of the Divining Rod*, although naturally the interpretations of dowsing then possible were less enlightened than they would have been with the benefit of today's scientific knowledge.

Even though it was realized that it was impossible to explain dowsing in purely physical terms, surprisingly little research was done, which led a leading dowser of the 1950s to admit that there hadn't been any major advances in the subject for thirty years.

Medical dowsing, called radiesthesia after the French word for it, started at about the turn of the century in France. Two French priests, the Abbés Bouley and Mermet, and other expert dowsers, Turenne, Lesourd and Bovis for example, were all beginning to appreciate the potential for medical dowsing. Abbé Mermet, for example, developed considerable expertise using a pendulum for dowsing and his book *Principles and Practice of Radiesthesia*, containing records of his results over a forty year period, became a classic in its day. The most important facet of his work was that he started to apply quantitative techniques which elevated a rather haphazard art into more of a science. It wasn't until 1939 though that knowledge of this application for dowsing came to England when the Medical Society for the Study of Radiesthesia was founded by Dr Guyon Richards. He surrounded himself with a group of interested and able doctors and lay people but the Society has all but died out today except for one notable member of the original group, Dr George Laurence, who has carried on the work and developed the techniques considerably. George Laurence, a skilled surgeon of his day, had become increasingly dissatisfied with orthodox medicine and what it could offer the vast numbers of patients with degenerative and untreatable ailments. 'We did not know the "why",' he said, 'and were reduced to treating names and labels, signs and symptoms, without a clue to causation; and hence the temporary alleviation of symptoms was the best that I, or any of my contemporaries, could do.'

He found his answer in radiesthesia and set about the job of linking homoeopathic remedies with radiesthetic diagnoses. The rules he laid down have now been used by many doctors for twenty-five years for the treatment of many chronic and supposedly incurable diseases.

The use of radiesthesia in medicine has been extended as a new science – psionic medicine (see page 246), but this embraces other medical philosophies too and is not simply medical dowsing. In 1968 the Psionic Medical Society was formed in Britain to encourage and foster a new approach to the science and art of healing. This Society was formed mainly for doctors but lay people were welcome to join as associate members.

But medical dowsing wasn't just catching on in Europe. Dr Albert Abrams, described by Sir James Barr as 'by far the greatest genius the medical profession has produced for half a century', produced, after an enormous amount of research, a 'black box'. From his original famous box came others, the Drown instruments and those of De-la-warr, all of which brought a new dimension to radiesthesia – the use of instruments for diagnosis and treatment. The use of instruments for this purpose became known as Radionics (see page 276). Unfortunately, even after the formation of the Radionic Association in 1943, thinking was still very bound by orthodox physics. Early radionics wallowed in gadgetry for its own sake and little progress was made. So little progress was being made that it led a distinguished dowser of the day, Mr W. O. Wood, to say at the Annual General Meeting of the British Society of Dowsers in 1955, 'The most important feature is the dowser's apparent unwillingness to tackle the full scope of the gift of sensitivity and his tendency to restrict his thoughts to what has been described as the hewing of wood and the drawing of water. The thinking public are now well aware that the range of sensitivity cannot thus be circumscribed. The problems facing mankind are greater than the locating of wells and matching of remedies – plumbing and plastering, so to speak – and we have to come to grips with the issues of our times and face realities as they are. It is necessary that the sights of the dowser be raised in line with those of science and philosophy – so a problem is presented: whether the urgency and magnitude of the factors facing man do not force upon the dowser the choice between widening the scope of his activities, or rejection as having failed to provide for the full flowering of the gift entrusted to him – for the principles the dowsers seek are known to others, who seek in turn the means of proving them. The dowser has the means of proving them, but appears these days to be blind to the principles.'

But slowly things did progress and as with so many areas of psychic research, Russia led the way. The Russians have built up an enormous body of research on radiesthesia and have used it for instance to find metals as deep as 240 feet under the ground. Today dowsing expertise is used all over the world for locating underground cables, conduits and pipes. Every major oil company has employed a dowser and cranked wires are on sale as 'pipe finders' in many a neighbourhood hardware store in the US.

How does it work?

We have to say in all honesty that nobody knows for sure but it is certainly a manifestation of a supersensory phenomenon and not simply a physical one. Dowsing, be it medical or not, needs the human being as an intermediary and some of us are naturally far better at it than others. In other words there's something in a human that acts as an amplifier of radiations of some kind arising from the substance being dowsed. It's important to realize though that there are two levels of dowsing. On one level, living and indeed non-living things (such as an underground river) give off some kind of radiation which can be picked up by a dowser. On quite another level, dead material and non-physical things can also be dowsed. It is on this second level (supersensible dowsing) that much of psionic and radionic medicine works.

As we saw in the Introduction, our paranormal senses can be educated and, fortunately for us, can be monitored too. Dowsing is a way of monitoring them. It is well known that under the right conditions our paranormal senses can produce involuntary muscular movements. Dowsing is exactly this. The receptive mind of the dowser causes his muscles to contract in ways quite beyond his control, so moving the rod, pendulum or whatever divining instrument he is using. Medical dowsers usually use a pendulum, as we shall see later, and with practice this provides clear answers to the questions in the operator's mind.

His mind though isn't simply the seat of his intellect. Indeed for all of us our minds are far more complex than simply the conjunction of consciousness and intellectual reasoning allows. Our minds only reason within the bounds of what our normal senses perceive but we have seen how limited this is. So the dowser's mind is affected not by his logical reasoning but by the supersensible forces that surround him. Of course it would be easy for him to override any movements he might feel himself making but he doesn't because part of his training is to cultivate a passivity that doesn't prejudge the outcome. This I found the most difficult to achieve in my few dalliances with a pendulum – it really does take a considerable degree of open-mindedness to be totally in the hands of the pendulum and the way it works.

Radiesthetists claim that all matter is associated with its own intrinsic energy fields in a form that the human body can pick up and register by means of a divining instrument. We know that water creates a very weak electromagnetic field in friction with soil, and many metals and metal ores in the earth's crust also have electromagnetic fields around them but radiesthetists go further than this. A Russian, Lakhowski, propounded the theory that every living cell vibrated or resonated with a sort of fundamental energy rather like a resonating electrical circuit with the energy circulating endlessly around the cell. He argued that when the cell is diseased or malfunctioning, the energy field around it changes and that this can be picked up. Most of us know that this is done using an ECG machine to detect abnormal heart muscle but, apart from similar measurements on muscles and brain cells, modern medicine hasn't done much to measure these electrical charges in other organs. The radiesthetist somehow 'locks on to' these minute energy changes (really they are simply modifications of the body's life forces) and can recognize them by the movement or change in movement of his dowsing equipment. At first I found this almost impossible to understand, let alone accept, but I can now see a possible way in which radiesthesia might work – and work it certainly does. The dowser is supersensitive to energy fields that come from his surroundings. This is partly because he is born with this skill and partly because he is aware of it and has developed it. The supersensible forces influence his body (it has been suggested that this occurs through the mass of body water that his body contains or through his blood) so as to modify the activity of his nervous system. This then makes his automatic (as opposed to his 'willed') nervous system do things quite beyond his control. In the majority of cases these changes in nervous control are picked up from his body and demonstrated to the outside world by the divining rod or pendulum he is holding.

At this time it is probably fruitless to concern ourselves any further with how dowsing works for work it certainly does and we are probably a very long way off being able to prove how anyway. Here are just a few proven uses of dowsing as listed in *The Dowsing Faculty* by Dr A. T. Westlake.

1. In the search for water, oil and mineral deposits.
2. In architecture. Some architects use dowsers in site selection, searching for cavities, pipes, drains, rivers and so on. It is said that certain susceptible people will never sleep well in a house built over an underground stream. This can be avoided by siting the house properly. Good dowsers can perform their skill simply by dowsing a map of the area – they don't even have to walk over the ground.
3. The location of missing property, dead bodies and missing persons, or archaeological remains.
4. Agricultural and horticultural uses. Here dowsing has a use in selecting optimum soil conditions, plant health and seed fertility. Foods too can be screened with a pendulum to show if they are wholesome.

5. Dr Oscar Brunler discovered a method of personality assessment which has industrial and educational potential, based on radiesthesia.

6. In homoeopathy radiesthesia is a great help in the selection of remedies – often a difficult problem (See later and also Psionic Medicine, page 246.)

7. The detection of low levels of pollutants including radioactivity otherwise unmeasurable by modern equipment.

8. Medical and veterinary uses.

9. Other uses. One medical radiesthetist I know is employed by a second-hand car dealer to divine the presence of rust that has been painted over and patched up before the sale or to determine the state of the engine without driving the car. His remarkable results are clearly of value to the car dealer.

How is it done?

A radiesthetist is a medical dowser – he may be medically trained but need not necessarily be. Radiesthesia is still in its infancy and is frankly frowned upon in most countries by the medical establishment. Radiesthesia is really not like conventional western medicine but is more like homoeopathy. Each patient is diagnosed individually and a unique diagnosis arrived at. For this reason, as with homoeopathy, two people presenting with apparently exactly the same complaint will receive different treatments. This is because although the superficial similarities are great (headache, runny nose, rash, fever etc.) the *real* underlying causes are different and so need different treatments.

Radiesthetists usually use a pendulum as their basic instrument. This takes the place of the dowser's twig or coathanger. A pendulum is used because it is sensitive and accurate, can be made of different substances and can even be made hollow to contain a particular object. A good and experienced radiesthetist may have several pendulums which he'll use for different things. The operator works from a sample or witness supplied by the patient. This sample usually takes the form of a piece of hair, a nail clipping or a spot of blood on a filter paper but exceptionally able radiesthetists can work from a photograph or even from the handwriting of the individual being treated.

The sort of pendulum used in medical dowsing is usually small and with a short thread. The thread is held between the thumb and forefinger over a sample and the response noted. There are three things the pendulum can do. It can oscillate to and fro, or it can gyrate clockwise or anticlockwise. These movements or combinations of movements provide the answers to questions posed by the dowser. Practice soon shows which movement means what in any given individual. For instance, by holding the pendulum over a known copper coin, one could then ask the question, 'is this made of copper?' and watch what the pendulum does. After several repetitions of similar procedures one arrives at a response of the pendulum which can be readily interpretable as 'yes'. This is then a standard 'reply' to any question asked.

The use of the pendulum then entails asking the right question but this isn't as easy as it might seem because in order to ask questions you have to have a knowledge of the subject. For example, if you knew that your coin was made of metal, yet you had never heard of copper, you would never arrive at its composition by dowsing because you wouldn't be able to ask the right question. This is one reason why medically qualified dowsers are unhappy about many of the non-medically qualified ones because it's all very well to ask questions but one has to ask the right ones and a doctor is much more likely to know which these are.

It might seem from what I've said that using a pendulum is difficult or a skill vouchsafed to a few exceptionally gifted psychics. Nothing could be further from the truth. A past president of the Society of Dowsers (who might be thought if anything to want to put forward the idea that he and his colleagues had a special ability or skill of some kind) has said that 80 per cent of people can become reasonable dowsers if they want and that only 10 per cent of people are hopeless. As with so many extrasensory phenomena, women are on the whole more successful than men.

If you go to a radiesthetist he'll take a sample or witness of hair, nail, blood or saliva from you. He keeps this in his files and uses it in your absence to do all his tests on. Because a radiesthetist works from witnesses that can be sent through the post, this means that someone undergoing radiesthetic diagnosis and treatment need never actually see the practitioner although most would want to take some sort of medical history personally.

RADIESTHESIA CAN BE USED TO DIAGNOSE ANY CONDITION, ACCORDING TO LEADING PRACTITIONERS

The witness is used by the radiesthetist in two ways. First he has to arrive at a diagnosis. This he does by using reference samples of various diseases, bacteria and so on placed on a specially constructed diagram or on a metre long wooden rule. The patient's sample is placed at one end (usually the zero mark) and a standard sample or witness at the 100 cm mark. These standard witnesses are either tiny sections of animal organs preserved in alcohol or specially prepared standards called Turenne witnesses (after the distinguished French engineer who invented them). The radiesthetist then takes his pendulum and oscillates it over the rule, moving it up and down the length of the rule until it spontaneously changes its direction and oscillates across the rule. This gives a reading in centimetres which he can use to determine whether the standard sample at the end of the rule is in fact related to the patient's disease. Having calibrated his rule from experience so he knows that with his working conditions a normal, healthy person's reading would be say 38 cm along from his sample, the radiesthetist can then calculate whether the patient's response is up or down on this. If, with the patient's witness at the zero on the rule and a Turenne liver witness at the 100 mark, the pendulum oscillates at right angles to the rule at the 34 cm mark, then the chances are that the patient's liver is underactive. Clearly, this all takes a great deal of practice and time but once the equipment is set up in its pre-set orientation (east–west is usually best with the radiesthetist facing north or south) the results are highly reproducible.

So, after taking a clinical history, the radiesthetist knows which organs are most likely to be affected, puts them up on his rule (or a diagnostic triangle which serves the same function) and arrives at the affected organ. He may then replace the organ witness with a disease or bacterial witness and repeat the pendulum readings. So by now he has arrived radiesthetically (possibly even in the patient's absence) at a diagnosis. Next he turns to his list of homoeopathic remedies and possibly holding the patient's witness in his left hand swings the pendulum over a list of likely cures. Once more the pendulum oscillates violently over the best drug. He then goes to a cabinet of homoeopathic remedies stored in tiny vials made up in all the commonly used concentrations. He goes back to the rule and puts the remedy he proposes to use in the concentration he thinks from experience will give the best results on the 100 cm mark. The pendulum then tells him whether his choice was correct. If it was not, he selects another concentration of the remedy as indicated by the pendulum's activity. Within a very few minutes he'll have selected not only the right remedy but will know the dose the patient needs *at that moment.*

The patient then takes his homoeopathic remedy and hopefully recovers. I say homoeopathic remedy but a radiesthetist will be able to confirm (or otherwise) the suitability of a conventional drug for a patient's condition using exactly the same methods. Radiesthetists themselves however would rarely recommend drugs as we know them.

All this is very hard work and even with the short cuts that they develop with experience it takes a lot of time to arrive at an accurate diagnosis and treatment. It also may be very exhausting for the practitioner. One radiesthetist I know (who incidentally makes uncannily accurate diagnoses by swinging his pendulum while listening to the patient on the telephone) becomes completely exhausted in two hours of diagnosis and treatment. As with most supersensible phenomena it takes a lot out of the practitioner who then needs to recharge his batteries.

The most astounding part of the whole procedure to me as a doctor is not that radiesthetists can do what they do but that the patient's witness, which may be several years old, can reflect what is happening in that patient in a dynamic way. Once a patient has sent a witness, the radiesthetist uses it time and time again to assess the success or otherwise of the therapy he's using and even to make new diagnoses. One lay radiesthetist I know will take out a patient's witness while he is on the telephone and without any information from the patient tell him what it is he is phoning about.

Clearly such a strange and uncanny medical practice has its enemies. In the USA radiesthesia is prohibited and in Belgium radiesthetists must by law use the patient directly and not a witness by itself. This law is sensible because patients treated at a distance can produce 'normal' readings to the radiesthetist yet be physically worse. In the UK there are hundreds of people, doctors and laymen, using this method of diagnosis and treatment selection but how long they will remain practising is under some doubt because new regulations to bring Britain in line with other EEC countries are likely within the next two years. This will not stop radiesthesia being practised but will drive it underground as in the USA.

Conventional medicine is unlikely to be able to accept this kind of practitioner for some time because as one leading *medical* radiesthetist puts it: 'There is something in medical education which turns you off any sort of unorthodox medicine and the trouble is that with any extrasensory perception phenomenon a sceptical climate is a bad one.' Things are changing though and with a broadening of medical horizons it could be that radiesthesia will at least be seriously considered by the medical establishment in the next decade or two.

What is it used for?

Radiesthesia can be used to diagnose any condition according to leading practitioners. After all, it is simply a method of arriving at a diagnosis and treatment using the human being as the diagnostic instrument. Many good intuitive doctors say that this is what they are doing all the time anyway. The pendulum is simply an outward manifestation and some highly gifted dowsers (either of medical or non-medical things) don't need to use a pendulum at all. So radiesthesia can, in the right hands, detect disease. Unfortunately we now come to the greatest crunch of all – the fact that radiesthetists claim to detect disease long before we doctors even dream anything is wrong with the patient. Medical science can only detect barn door differences and changes in the human state and can't detect changes in the higher spiritual planes or energy forces of the body at all. Radiesthetists claim to pick up changes in the etheric or supersensible body extremely early, long before the disease processes causing them have become irreversible or even detectable in the physical body. This in fact, if it is a justifiable claim, is where radiesthetists should be able to help us in the future. Today's methods by and large diagnose disease when it is too late to cure it. Certainly we can reduce symptoms and even sometimes reverse things temporarily but by and large, by the time a doctor can measure something, the damage is done. Radiesthesia may well be able to pick up disease processes much earlier and so allow treatment to be started sooner. If this were to be the case, as many medically trained and highly responsible radiesthetists I know claim, then we would be able to provide a *health* service instead of a *sickness* service – and that would be some advance!

But having said this, it makes radiesthesia almost impossible to assess in our classical medical terms because, if they're claiming to treat people in whom we cannot even detect disease, how can we possibly tell whether they're doing any good? Also, as with homoeopathy and many of the other fringes of medicine, the fact that every individual is treated in a unique way means that one can never do controlled trials. Even if they were possible it is unlikely they'd be done by radiesthetists themselves who know only too well that their treatments work and who are too busy treating people to take years off to study *why* they're successful. Anyway, they argue, even if it were mumbo-jumbo they can't do any harm simply because they use only homoeopathic remedies which according to the same medical sceptics have no effect anyway. Valuable time can be wasted when a patient with a potentially treatable condition goes to a radiesthetist instead of to his doctor but this is happening all the time in our present health care system so the rare occasions on which it happens in radiesthetic practice shouldn't concern anyone too much.

What of the future?

The near future looks as bad for radiesthesia as the long term looks good in my opinion. As we come to realize that it might be another way of arriving at the same end point as conventional medicine, it could be regarded with less hostility but the vast majority of doctors in the medical establishment is light years away from accepting the use of extrasensory perception in the diagnosis and treatment of disease.

Anyway, radiesthetists say, there's very little chance that it could catch on in a big way even if it were shown to be of great value tomorrow, simply because so few people have the ability to use a pendulum at this level of expertise and so few are sensitive to the supersensible world of which radiesthesia is a part. It is a difficult subject to teach except to another sensitive and able (in the psychic sense) person and most people would find it too arduous personally to perform on a daily basis. It could never be as simple as prescribing a drug or tonic which requires very little effort indeed on the practitioner's behalf and a proportion of these easily dispensed 'goodies' do in fact work.

As with homoeopathy and many of the patient-centred fringes of medicine, the time taken to assess and treat the patient wouldn't be workable in our current health care system. In the long term though such fringe medical disciplines could save enormous amounts of time, money and suffering.

Radionics

Definition

A therapy that has grown up around the ability of the human being to use radiesthesia together with simple instruments to help in the diagnosis of disease in animals, plants and humans and then to treat this disease at a distance without the presence of the patient.

Background

Radionics is more akin to spiritual healing than anything else and has come in for a lot of criticism mainly because it uses 'magic boxes' and claims to be a science in its own right. Slowly but surely radionics is catching on but the orthodox medical profession can't accept it on a wide scale and it is still illegal in most states in the USA.

The story starts at the turn of the century when an American physician, Dr Albert Abrams, described by Sir James Barr, a past President of the British Medical Association, as 'by far the greatest genius the medical profession has produced for half a century', discovered that a patient of his with cancer of the lip had a small area of dullness on his abdomen when it was percussed. Doctors use percussion (the tapping of the middle finger of the left hand with the tip of the middle finger of the right hand while the former is in contact with the body) to detect areas of dullness or resonance. This is an ancient skill and very helpful in diagnosis. What Abrams discovered though was that only when his cancer patient was facing west was he able to elicit a change in percussion note over a well-defined area of his abdominal wall. He soon became enthused with the possibilities of such a diagnostic system and assembled patients suffering from all kinds of disease. Facing them all due west he percussed them and found characteristic areas of dullness on specific areas of the body. Needless to say, as a man of scientific integrity, he repeated all these experiments with normal people – with no sign of any dull areas.

The next stage in his experiments was a momentous one. He took a small container, placed it on the forehead of a fit, healthy man and then placed a piece of malignant tumour in the container. On percussion of the man's abdomen he found an area of dullness just as he had found with the real cancer patients in the past. In other words, a piece of diseased tissue placed in contact with a healthy person altered his nervous system in such a way as to change the percussion note in the abdomen. This experiment was the birth of radionic diagnosis.

He then went on to suggest that diseased tissue might be radiating an abnormal wave form of some kind which influenced the healthy man in some way. Since he and the other early experimenters thought these waves might be radio waves, the science was called 'radionics'. He designed experiments with samples of diseased tissues behind a screen and an electrode, connected to the healthy subject's forehead, joined to a wire which led behind the screen. Abrams percussed systematically while an assistant, unseen by him, took the end of the wire connected to the man's head and placed it over various diseased tissues in turn. He soon found that he could tell exactly which diseased tissue was being 'sampled' by his assistant simply by the area of the body that became dull to percussion. Unfortunately, it soon became apparent that cancer and syphilis both produced dullness in the same area of the abdomen and Abrams had to find a way of distinguishing the two.

Electronics was in its infancy at the time, yet with a good knowledge of electricity and the help of some very good apparatus (Abrams was a very rich man by inheritance and so could afford such luxuries to experiment with) he was able to construct a box with a variable resistance in it. He then found that cancer and syphilis produced a dullness over the same area of the abdomen but that cancer would only do so with a 50 ohm resistance in the wire and syphilis with a 55 ohm resistance. Over years of painstaking research he found that he didn't need actual pieces of diseased tissue in order to get these results – but that he could produce exactly similar and reproducible results using a spot of blood absorbed on to a piece of filter paper. By devising more and more sophisticated resistance circuits, he was able to make finer and finer distinctions between diseased tissues and eventually perfected the equipment to a stage where he could tell which of several people had *touched* a piece of paper (even hours before). He proposed therefore that these pieces of paper, blood spots or whatever had retained what he termed 'human energy' for hours or even longer.

News of all this soon spread and doctors flocked to him from all over his native America and from Europe. Abrams constructed equipment and sold it to qualified doctors whom he instructed in its use. It's easy to feel sceptical about such an invention today but remember this was long before any 'wonder drugs' and doctors could offer very little by way of positive help to many of their patients.

But as with many a discovery there was scepticism, jealousy and disbelief among the worthies of the day. In 1922 a group was set up under the chairmanship of Sir Thomas (later Lord) Horder to investigate these magic black boxes. In the first test, twenty-five successive trials were successful and one of the team calculated that the odds against this happening by chance were 1 in 33,554,432! The members of the Royal Society of Medicine in London weren't sure whether they should even listen to a report on such a cranky subject but in the end they decided to do so. They heard all the evidence and came to the conclusion that although the fundamental propositions underlying radionics were 'established to a very high degree of probability . . . there does not appear to be any sanction for this kind of practice at the present time'.

With the death of Abrams and the spread of ill-informed criticism, most doctors were discouraged from taking the research further but good ideas don't lie down and die that easily. Radionics could have died though but for the pioneering work of Ruth Drown, an American chiropractor. She has three radionic firsts to her credit. She was the first to treat people at a distance; the first to realize the importance of the endocrine glands in radionics; and the first to take photographs of the internal organs of her patients. She also developed and modified Abrams' equipment to make it more sensitive and therefore more useful but we don't have space to go into the details here.

Because she was so confident (as most pioneers have to be to get anything done against a sceptical background), she was led to take on more patients than she could easily handle and after a while someone complained that her methods were useless as far as he was concerned. Whether or not there was any truth in this, it gave the medical profession and the American Food and Drug Administration just the excuse they were looking for to nail radionics for good.

In Drown's trial in 1951 numerous people came forward to testify that her methods had cured them and when the jury went out to consider its verdict the court stenographer was convinced that she'd be acquitted. However, the jury was obviously very swayed by the radio experts who testified that the results could not possibly be achieved by radio waves (which is what early radionics practitioners thought the radiations from living matter were) and Ruth Drown was convicted of fraud and medical quackery and sent to jail in the early sixties after years of appeals. In the interim the authorities seized and destroyed all her instruments. When she finally emerged from jail she suffered a stroke and died soon after.

Once more radionics suffered a near mortal blow but other workers in England were not being so overtly silenced and good research was also under way in the USSR. Dr Guyon Richards in England was a dogged researcher who found to his amazement 'that the atomic numbers of the elements corresponded to the figures on my rheostats when I was tuning in on my circuits; that is, hydrogen, the first element, caused a reflex on 1 ohm, oxygen on 8 ohms, sodium on 11, sulphur on 16 and so on . . .' He also did considerable work on the auras that psychics can see around people or that can be seen by many people when using a Kilner screen (see page 147). He was probably the first person to realize the value of radionics as a tool in the detection of disease *before* it had become clinically apparent, by discovering that the force fields around the body are altered in pre-disease states and not only when the body is seriously ill. This facet of radionics remains until today one of the great advantages it has over all other forms of medicine.

The last great step forward for radionics was taken by George 'Bill' de la Warr, an English engineer. He and a small team tried to refine and improve upon the work of Abrams and Drown and built up a substantial worldwide reputation for radionics. It was De la Warr and his wife who set out to standardize the equipment right from scratch in an effort to make the results of radionic instruments as reproducible and scientific as possible. Over years of experimentation they found that seven out of ten people could operate their diagnostic instruments to some extent and of these three could do so extremely well. They tried, with some success, to make radionics respectable and encouraged doctors to work with them. De la Warr invented a very special camera with which he took some 12,000 photographs of the blood spots of his patients. These photographs gave information about the internal conditions of the patients. For example, one woman living 200 miles away from his laboratory sent a blood spot with a request that he check on her pregnancy and tell her when to expect the child. A series of photographs were produced using the 'life force energies' from the blood spot that allowed De la Warr to make some very helpful predictions. A doctor at a leading hospital (both of which have to remain secret to this very day) borrowed this extraordinary camera from De la Warr and took 400 photographs of samples from patients at his hospital. Medical pressure made him get rid of the camera but he maintained that it had been very useful. He quoted an example of a woman with a suspected advanced brain tumour. He put her blood spot on the camera and tuned it to the setting on the camera representing brain tumour. When the plate was developed it showed a cross section of a skull with a large tumour. Autopsy soon after confirmed the picture exactly. 'Nobody', commented the doctor, 'could possibly have faked the picture – they simply wouldn't have had the anatomical knowledge.'

The De la Warrs formed the Radionic Centre Organization in 1965 (the name was changed to the Radionic and Magnetic Centre Organization in 1970) and continued to do remarkable research including a link up between a young man in Oxford, England, and his photograph in New York. In the presence of impartial witnesses, some from the Government, the photograph placed in a radionic instrument in New York promptly caused alterations on a plotting machine connected to the young man whose photo it was in Oxford. This stunning experiment didn't help explain *how* radionics worked though and it is this difficulty in explaining how it works that remains the greatest bar to its acceptance today. The De la Warrs too were taken to court but the judge dismissed every allegation of fraud. In fact, so impressive was the array of distinguished witnesses that it acted as a public testament to radionics. For nine years after this ordeal De la Warr continued in productive work until he died in 1969. Much of the new thinking now comes from two British practitioners, Malcolm Rae and David Tansley.

How is it done?

The exact technique involved in radionics varies according to the instrument being used but they all have certain features in common. I'll describe here the use of the De la Warr instrument.

The sample or witness used is usually a spot of the patient's blood on a piece of filter paper but it could be a piece of hair or nail. The device contains a small bar magnet that is rotated to 'tune' the whole instrument with the 'field wave' of the patient's sample. There is a series of dials on which a specific frequency is set for the condition under scrutiny. There is also a control dial to show the degree of severity of the condition being studied. Lastly there is a cavity covered with a rubber membrane that gives a 'yes' or 'no' answer to a mentally posed question by the operator. The way this is used is that when posing a question, the operator pulls his fingers repeatedly across the membrane until a 'yes' response is obtained to a particular question asked. When the answer is 'yes', friction increases between the fingers and the membrane and the fingers seem to 'stick'. This stick method of defining the end point is simply another manifestation of the radiesthetic faculty and is said to be brought about by a tiny increase in sweat production of the operator's fingers when he is asking the right question. Other instruments use a pendulum to determine this end point but it doesn't matter which is used because they both simply record a change in the operator's involuntary nervous system when he 'tunes' into the right question.

So with the patient's witness in a well on the device and the magnet tuned to the patient's 'frequency' (as determined radiesthetically), the operator takes a written list of the patient's most troublesome symptoms and with all the dials of the device at zero uses a probe to touch each question in turn while holding the mentally held question, 'Is this the main symptom?' As the pendulum or 'stick' membrane gives him the answers, he follows this with more precise mental questions until he has run the diseased organ or diseased process to earth.

The dials are used to tune the instrument so as to register the degree of deviation of the patient's sample from the healthy norm. The radionic practitioner thinks of the perfect functioning of the organ he's concerning himself with and measures with his dial the discrepancy between this and reality as represented by the energy emanating from the blood spot in the well. The instrument is continuously adjusted from the perfect setting (which has previously been worked out for each organ and is kept as a standard) by slow rotation of the balance dial until the practitioner becomes aware of the new balance between the instrument and the patient. At this point he can read off the actual degree of imbalance. He becomes aware of the new balance point either by a change in stickiness of the rubber pad or by using a pendulum (see page 268).

Once the diagnosis is made there are two major ways in which treatment can be administered. First, the treatment can be arrived at radiesthetically by asking the right mental questions or by using a pendulum over treatment tables. The substance required by the patient at that particular stage is thus arrived at. This can then be given as a homoeopathic remedy direct to the patient or can be 'transmitted' by thought power to the patient who may be miles away. Just how this might work we shall soon see.

Radionic instruments are difficult for most people to understand. They contain no electrical circuitry as such and the vast majority are not mains powered. Radionics is really a branch of radiesthesia, as we have seen and as such it deals with the interaction between mind and matter. A really gifted American psychic healer and diagnostician such as Edward Cayce, perhaps the most gifted psychic of this kind, could, with incredible reliability, diagnose and treat people at great distances by thought power alone. Although *this* power of healing thought is found only in a tiny number of people, many others can achieve the same results but less reliably and less often. This is probably because most of us simply can't concentrate single-mindedly on the healing we're involved in. It was because of this that radionic instruments were invented. They enable people with very low psychic abilities to produce good results and to reproduce them at a later date. Once the basic pattern of either the patient's illness or the necessary therapy is established, by resetting the dials on the device to the same readings, the practitioner can take over where he left off previously and if necessary transmit the same treatment in a predictable way. Eventually, it should be possible for a practised radionic operator to do away with his instruments entirely but few people are capable of doing this and so stay with their tangible prop – just as doctors still order laboratory tests even if they're quite happy about the diagnosis and treatment they're pursuing.

A radionic analysis is not the same as a medical diagnosis because the doctor is looking for disease, whereas the radionic practitioner is looking for underlying causes. The main problem with radionics in non-medical hands is that the right questions may not be asked and so the operator will never arrive at the right answer. Unfortunately he might arrive at the wrong answer by misinterpreting the answer or by asking a slightly erroneous question. To be fair though, this can happen in orthodox medicine.

How does it work?

Nobody knows for sure and this is one of the major stumbling blocks to the wider acceptance of radionics. It's certain that it doesn't work by radio waves as the early pioneers thought.

Leading practitioners today such as Malcolm Rae have begun to concentrate on the 'how' now that they no longer need to prove that radionics works. Rae uses a helpful analogy to explain the link between thought and geometrical expression (which is what the dials on a radionic apparatus produce). When a composer thinks of a tune, he expresses it as notes on a score. The orchestra plays these notes and a gramophone record is made of the performance. The geometrical patterns (undulations in the record's groove) are thus to all intents and purposes storing the original thoughts of the composer in a readily accessible form. So it is with a radionic instrument. By working out the 'rate' or setting of the dials for a given disease or treatment the pattern is stored as a thought process and it is this thought process that is used in treatment.

Radionics is beyond explanation in terms of conventional physics or medicine – it doesn't conform to scientific laws we accept today and as such has to be explained in rather unusual language. As we saw in the Introduction (see page 30), all matter is composed of atoms and at the sub-atomic level all matter is notional and can only be expressed in terms of energy. Harold Burr first discovered electromagnetic body fields around humans (some of which are measurable using instruments sensitive to electromagnetic energy) but also found that there were other fields at a distance from the body that were not electromagnetic in nature. As more research is done it seems to show that when it comes to electrical fields we are like a set of Russian dolls, each having another smaller one inside it. An energy field is difficult to define even in modern terms but can be expressed as that which connects two events in space in the absence of any visible connection.

So all life is really a collection of sophisticated energy fields. Burr's great discovery was that disease disrupted these life fields and did so even before any visible or medically measurable disease was present. Abrams himself had diagnosed a cancer in his own seemingly well wife radionically a full ten years before she died of it! A pupil of Burr, Dr Leonard J. Ravitz Jr, had done considerable research to show that the mind can alter these energy fields, so it is easy to understand how anxiety, grief or worry really can alter the body physically. This disorganization caused by mental processes is probably the basis for psychosomatic illness.

Radionics then looks like working on the same basis as thought transfer. The Russians have an enormous literature on thought transfer. Professor Vasiliev of Leningrad University has conducted well-authenticated demonstrations of thought transfer over a distance of 900 miles. Malcolm Rae, the English radionics expert, has successfully treated people by thought patterns magnetically energized, regardless of distance, and this possibility is a common experience of many absent healers and radionic practitioners.

So it seems that thought at one point in time and space can influence patients at quite another point in space instantaneously and with no visible connection. This leads us to the inescapable conclusion that thought acts like an energy field. Edward W.

Russell, an American journalist, whose book *Report on Radionics* is about the most sensible thing written on the subject, proposes certain new fields in order that we can understand the processes going on. After decades of studying radionics and getting to know many of the key figures, he proposes the existence of what he calls T-fields (short for thought fields). These are not electromagnetic fields and can't be measured by any method known to Man except by Man's own body. T-fields exist quite apart from the human brain, which is a 'computer' of great power and sophistication, but only that. Just as a computer is quite distinct from the information stored in it, so T-fields or thought waves are nothing to do with the brain as such. They simply reside in brain cells in preference to other things but can latch on to other things too. This is well demonstrated in the power of psychometry. Some sensitive people can, with uncanny accuracy, describe past events associated with an object (or part of it) simply by holding it. They can read out the memory held in the object.

As far as we know, thought waves can traverse space and are not affected by time. Russell goes on to propose that in addition to T-fields there are other fields that are Nature's 'master blueprints' for all matter. These he calls O-fields (O for organizing). These O-fields control the very nature of matter and are distinct from thought fields which are created by us and function in the context of human knowledge and memory. So on this basis the patient's witness puts the overall organizing field of the practitioner in touch with the patient's O-field. Once the two O-fields are linked, it doesn't matter how far apart the two people are. There is instant communication between the two. No one knows how this is actually achieved in the practitioner's body but somehow the O-field changes the working of his autonomic nervous system in such a way as to cause his finger to stick on a pad, alter the behaviour of a pendulum or, as in Abrams's experience, change abdominal resonance, detectable by percussion.

Edgar Cayce had a direct and extremely rare connection

between his O-field and his brain. Whilst asleep he would dictate to his secretary all the details of his patient who was miles away. We have all heard of doctors who have uncannily accurate hunches about patients and I have personally known instinctively what is wrong with patients on numerous occasions. This also explains how it is that a mother knows that something has befallen her child even when the child is far away and perhaps helps answer the riddle of identical twins and their often-reported powers of knowing what each other is doing. Perhaps they share an O-field?

So in summary, radionics, dowsing and radiesthesia all possibly work by thought transfer between O-fields. It will be decades before we can prove any of this in terms that modern science will find acceptable but in the meantime we might as well accept the theory as the best we have to explain a remarkable phenomenon.

Reflexology

Definition

An ancient Chinese and Indian diagnostic and therapeutic system in which the soles of the feet and less commonly the palms of the hands are massaged deeply.

Background

Probably about the same time that acupuncture was first flourishing in Ancient China, reflexology was born. It was almost unknown in the West though until the beginning of this century, when an American ear, nose and throat specialist, Dr William H. Fitzgerald, created an interest in the subject, which he called zone therapy as had the Chinese in 3000 BC who used it in conjunction with acupuncture. He found that by pressing firmly or massaging certain areas of the body, effects were produced in other, quite distant parts.

The greatest single exponent of this science in the West was another American – Eunice D. Ingham – who developed Fitzgerald's teachings in the 1930s and came to concentrate almost exclusively on the feet zones. Because she did so much for the technique, it is sometimes called the Ingham Reflex Method of Compression Massage. Today, reflexology is growing in popularity and there are hundreds of practitioners in the West, the majority of whom are in the USA. Most of the top practitioners today learned from Ingham herself and schools have grown up in England, Belgium and France. Many reflexologists are already involved in another form of natural therapy such as osteopathy, homoeopathy or chiropractic.

Most people immediately imagine that reflexology must be something to do with chiropody but this is not so. Certainly, some physical diseases of the foot can cause stimulation of the reflex zones and cause symptoms and signs to appear elsewhere (for example an ingrowing toenail can produce headaches) but this is not the real basis of reflexology. The nature of chiropody is rather different and involves surgical techniques to cure and prevent diseases of the feet. Reflexology uses the feet to prevent and cure disease *in the rest of the body*.

How is it done?

The patient is asked to lie on a comfortable couch with both feet uncovered. The reflexologist then gently feels over them and by locating the sites of 'crystalline' or 'gritty' substances deep under the skin can diagnose which organs are affected by disease. A reflexologist 'reads' the feet like a blind person reads Braille until these crystals are found. As he presses over them, the patient feels pain in the area pressed; in the area of the body represented there; and sometimes in both places. The degree of pain experienced in the foot can be extreme, even if the reflexologist simply strokes the surface of the skin over the reflex point very gently. Because of this extreme sensitivity, many reflexologists only stroke the skin when treating the old or the very young for fear of producing too much pain.

Treatments consist of pressure applied with the edge of the thumb or finger, rotated clockwise. The pressure is usually quite deep but need not be painful. A good reflexologist would rather repeat many short, pain-free treatments than go all out to cure the malady in a single painful treatment. Each session lasts from ten to thirty minutes and several sessions may be needed. Often though the complaint clears up after a single treatment session.

Patients' reactions to the treatment vary but sometimes the body reacts violently while the disordered system is righting itself. Some patients feel emotionally shattered and others feel invigorated by the treatment.

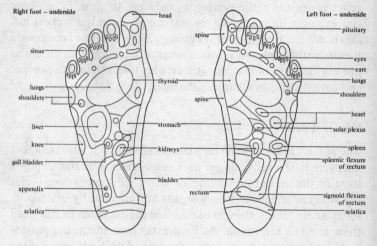

Right foot – underside

head
sinus
lungs
shoulders
liver
knee
gall bladder
appendix
sciatica
thyroid
stomach
kidneys
bladder
spine

Left foot – underside

pituitary
spine
eyes
ears
lungs
shoulders
heart
solar plexus
spleen
spleenic flexure
of rectum
sigmoid flexure
of rectum
sciatica
rectum

Diagrams showing the organs of the body as represented on the feet

What is it used for?

Reflexology, like acupuncture, is most successful with functional disorders. It's unlikely that it will cure a raging infection and it can certainly do nothing for structural abnormalities such as hernias, obstruction of the bowel or a broken leg. Reflexologists seem to get good results with constipation, asthma, stress states, bladder trouble, headaches and even more dramatic conditions such as kidney- and gall-stones. Migraine does especially well with reflexology and sinus trouble can also be quickly alleviated.

Over the period of one treatment session, or over several sessions, the pains in the particular reflex points slowly disappear as the body's own healing forces correct the physiological imbalances.

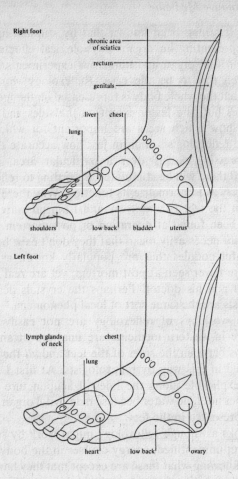

Right foot

chronic area of sciatica

rectum

genitals

liver chest

lung

shoulders   low back   bladder   uterus

Left foot

lymph glands of neck   chest

lung

heart   low back   ovary

How does it work?

It is well known by modern medicine that the internal organs are represented on the surface of the body by areas of skin that share the same nerve supplies as these organs. A condition affecting the diaphragm, for instance, will often present as pain in the shoulder tip, simply because both share the same nerve supply. It has long been known that by stimulating the skin surface representing an organ, physiological effects could be produced in that organ and numerous experiments in animals have proven this to be the case. Reflexology works on the principle that the whole body is represented on the feet – mostly on the soles but to a lesser extent on the sides and tops. The diagrams show which areas are important for which internal organs and reflexologists confirm just how accurate these areas are. By pressing deeply over a particular area, the organ represented there will be stimulated, according to reflexologists, in such a way as to normalize its function. Why there should be 'crystals' in the feet I cannot say and I am unaware that they have ever been found at operation or post mortem. However, this need not necessarily mean that they don't exist because the hard, painful nodules that are popularly known as 'fibrositic nodules' are never seen at post mortem, yet are real enough to the patient and his doctor. Perhaps the crystals described by reflexologists are the same sort of local phenomena.

But the workings of reflexology are not easily explained because we in western medicine are unaware of any nervous connections between the soles of the feet and *all* the areas said to be linked in this way by reflexologists. At first I thought it might be explicable along the lines of acupuncture meridians but that does not hold water because many vital organ meridians are not represented in the feet.

So it looks as though reflexology might work by stimulating other, as yet unidentified, energy courses in the body. We have no way of knowing what these are except that they have real and reproducible functional effects in the body.

Rolfing

Definition

A body therapy, more accurately called structural integration, invented by an American, Ida Rolf.

Background

Ida Rolf graduated in biological chemistry from Barnard College, New York, in 1920 and soon became interested in health problems. Quite how she developed her therapy isn't known but by the 1940s people were seeking her help and presumably obtaining relief. She worked for thirty-five years without recognition until the mid-sixties when, with the enormous growth of interest in the human potential movement, her message began to catch on in a big way.

In the past twelve years, she has trained over 150 rolfers and more than 55,000 people in Mexico, Germany, Israel, Canada, the USA, England and India have been rolfed. In 1970 Ida Rolf set up the Rolf Institute of Structural Integration in Boulder, Colorado, to train practitioners, sponsor research and act as an information centre on rolfing.

How does it work?

Rolfing is a kind of deep massage which manipulates the tissues of the body in such a way as to break down connective tissue that shouldn't be there. Rolf's basis for the therapy lies in the fact that most of us in the western world have poor posture caused by our physical and psychological environments. So that the body can maintain these abnormal postures, the muscles of certain areas are thrown into unnatural contraction, thus encouraging the connective tissues in the area to overgrow to form thickened plates which further restrict natural movement and posture.

Imagine a plumb line running through the ear, shoulder, pelvis and ankle bone. If a person's head hangs forward of this line it will be outside the downward vertical force of gravity and will have to be held in position by exceptional activity in the neck muscles, which are thus working overtime. As the years go by, the body's response to repeated strain on a muscle not only builds up the *muscle* itself but also causes the formation of other connective tissues in the body known as fascia.

We all have fascia running as connective bands and sheaths all over our bodies but medical science has never considered it to be a dynamic or changing substance. Rolfers maintain that, by freeing these thickened, fibrous bands of tissue, the body can be loosened up and then structurally re-ordered slightly to improve posture and indeed the person's whole well-being.

How is it done?

First, the rolfer carefully observes the rolfee in his or her underwear, looking for abnormalities in posture and unnatural tension. The rolfee is then photographed from the front, back and side to document this starting point. After each of ten sessions the rolfee is photographed again and any changes noted.

Each session lasts one hour and the rolfee lies on a table while the rolfer pushes deeply and slides across the skin surface. The rolfer releases thickened and stuck fascia by pressure with hands, elbows, knuckles and fingers and by carefully using his body weight can exert considerable force if needed. This process is repeated for seven one-hour sessions which concentrate in turn on a major area such as the head, chest, pelvis and so on. The last three sessions 're-integrate' the body segments after the first seven have loosened them up.

Rolfees report a feeling of deep pressure and even excruciating pain on occasions as the treatment is carried out. Some say they feel 'lighter' or talk of a trembling all over the body. Others say they feel an increased awareness which leads to a fresh outlook on life. Pain seems to be a fairly common and unpleasant feature of the treatment but it is soon forgotten when the rolfee gets up and feels so much better. Ida Rolf is annoyed at the emphasis put on the painful aspect of the therapy. 'The pain of psycho-therapy is just as great as that of rolfing . . . and it's just as disorganizing in the beginning,' she says. 'They particularly get pains if they resist the process. The way to get off the pains is to go into the pain, to make it as tough as you know how and all of a sudden it isn't there.'

The pleasure or pain sensed also depends on the emotions linked to the part being rolfed. Rolf tells of a man who panicked every time she got near his neck. He had the sensation that he was drowning. After this sensation had passed he described how he nearly drowned when three years old and was revived by resuscitation. Rolf feels that this kind of psychological re-awakening and coming to terms with possibly unpleasant things in the past is all a valuable, though not essential, part of her method. Undoubtedly rolfing is the sort of therapy that means different things to different people. To some it is simply a kind of super physiotherapy and to others a stimulus for mental self-adjustment too.

The remarkable thing about rolfing is that those who are rolfed actually get taller (by half an inch or so) as borne out by 'before and after' photographs. The ten hour treatment course brings about permanent postural improvement and photographs taken of people who have been rolfed as long as ten years before still show elongation of their bodies. Increased comfort and suppleness is something these rolfees also comment on.

It is said that Cary Grant, Georgia O'Keeffe and Greta Garbo have been rolfed and it is undoubtedly catching on in the USA generally. Ida Rolf doesn't just rolf people though – she has had good results with many different kinds of animals including race horses. Other rolfers are trying its benefits on autistic and cerebral palsied (spastic) children but it's early days to say just how good the results will be.

Why does it work?

Undoubtedly it is possible to break down fibrous connective tissue in the body if enough force is used. But to break down these tissues through the skin must mean that there'll be quite a lot of pain, especially as very often these overgrown tissues are attached to bone, the covering of which (the periosteum) is exquisitely tender if stretched or torn. Professor Valerie Hunt and Dr Wayne Massey of the University of California at Los Angeles' Movement Behavior EMG Laboratory designed special equipment to record and measure muscle responses in various activities performed before and after ten rolfing sessions. Their subjects were eleven healthy males between the ages of twenty-five and forty-five. They found from very sophisticated measurements of the electrical activities in the muscles that body movements were smoother, larger and less constrained; that body movements were more energetic; that there were fewer unnecessary movements; that their carriage was more erect and that there was less strain needed to maintain a good posture.

Other research is also under way to study the unnatural thickenings of fascia that rolfing is supposed to break down. Classical anatomical dissection pays little attention to the fascia but these new studies hope to prove beyond doubt that fascial thickenings are the underlying cause of the troubles cured by rolfing.

As with so many manipulative therapies it's difficult to know just how useful rolfing is compared with others. The Alexander Technique probably obtains some of the same results rolfing does but without pain and without any pretence of altering the structure of the body. A really good massage in capable hands has an invigorating effect, so how much of rolfing might simply be explained along these lines? Many people experience a renewed vigour and even an emotional catharsis during rolfing but, if it can have positive psychological effects, might it not also arouse emotions and dredge up tensions that are not helped by the technique?

Rolfing is undoubtedly a useful body therapy for some but its future depends on very much larger numbers of people experiencing it under controlled conditions and a lot more research.

Shiatsu

Definition

Literally finger pressure, Shiatsu is a form of oriental massage and pressure designed to stimulate the acupuncture points and meridians.

Background

Shiatsu is an ancient Japanese medical therapy which arose spontaneously and independently at about the same time as did acupuncture in China. It has always been a kind of family medicine in Japan, a remedial massage performed by one member of a family upon another. But behind this seemingly simple practice is an enormous amount of background knowledge and folklore.

How does it work?

Basically Shiatsu involves finger pressure over the acupuncture points and meridians. This is why it is also called (in the West) acupressure – or acupuncture without needles. One of the problems with acupuncture is that the practitioner has to be very expert at using his needles in order to obtain just the desired response. Shiatsu on the other hand, because it uses only the fingers, allows more leeway in terms of the area stimulated and also relieves the patient of any concern about unsterilized acupuncture needles. So, quite simply, Shiatsu works for the same reasons that acupuncture does (see page 73).

How is it done?

Shiatsu takes two forms. Either the patient is massaged firmly but painlessly over certain areas of his body in order to stimulate the flow of the body's energy patterns and so harmonize them, or otherwise a single fingertip of the therapist is used to stimulate specific acupuncture points.

Unlike rolfing (see page 293), Shiatsu is not painful. The massage and the pressure technique both stop short of producing pain but still act deeply on occasions. Some Shiatsu practitioners also use certain osteopathic and chiropractic techniques although this is almost certainly a western embellishment of the original Japanese therapy.

Shiatsu can be used prophylactically even if one is not actually ill but is also useful for specific disease conditions. Once learnt, many Shiatsu techniques can be helpful in a domestic situation (see Do-in) and there are many first-aid procedures in Shiatsu. I know a doctor who re-aligned the badly twisted and broken leg of a patient who was caught up a mountain in a skiing accident. The doctor had no anaesthetics or pain-killers, so he asked another skier to press over a Shiatsu point so as to leave him free to straighten and splint the broken leg. Some Shiatsu devotees never have a dental anaesthetic but simply press over the correct acupuncture point during the painful phases of the dental procedure.

Shiatsu is still enormously popular in Japan and is now catching on in the USA. There are probably 300–400 practitioners in the USA and in Europe about 500 people in Belgium alone have received benefit from Shiatsu. It is also gaining popularity in Holland.

A lot of Shiatsu is intuitive in all of us. The mother who rubs her child's abdomen when he has a tummy ache is stimulating the body's energy forces in much the same way that a Shiatsu practitioner does. It is simply a transfer of healing power from one person to another – a way of neutralizing energy patterns in the body that are out of alignment. In western medicine the nearest most of us have come to this is in the acceptance of remedial massage (that makes one feel better for reasons inexplicable in purely anatomical terms) and 'the hand on the fevered brow'. Many of us when ill will have noticed how much better we feel if a kindly and sympathetic person simply lays his hand upon our head, or indeed any affected part. The relief from pain and anguish can be dramatic but we cannot explain it in terms of western medicine. The orientals know exactly what is going on. They say that all these remedies carried out by the laying on of hands are a quite natural expression of our abilities to harmonize our vital energy fields with those of another person. Even the truly cynical have to admit they feel entirely different after as little as forty-five minutes of Shiatsu massage.

What is it used for?

Shiatsu can be used to prevent disease – simply to keep the body in harmony with the environment. Most of us live in a very unnatural environment today and we haven't adapted to it very well, especially when it comes to our food environment. Shiatsu practitioners almost always take the opportunity of re-educating their patients in matters of diet and most suggest a much more natural and old-fashioned diet which we in the West call macrobiotic (see page 198). Because so much of oriental medicine is firmly based on the understanding that disease comes from within (western medicine by and large believes that disease comes from outside the body), Shiatsu practitioners will go to great pains to improve the nutrition and general mental health of their patients by improving their life style. It is this, together with the Shiatsu technique itself, that makes their patients better.

Shiatsu can be used to alter the energy flows in the body either to tone them up or sedate them. A good Shiatsu practitioner can make the person feel elated or sedated depending on what he does and which meridians he stimulates. He uses the face as the mirror of the body and treats various parts according to what he sees in the face. Very often a patient will come to Shiatsu complaining of pains which western doctors have misinterpreted. For example, one practitioner I know sees lots of patients with so-called sciatica but he knows they don't in fact have it. The meridian that runs down the sciatic area links to the gall-bladder and often these 'sciatic' patients are relieved of their troubles by having their diseased gall-bladder removed. Western medicine simply wouldn't make this link. The Shiatsu practitioner re-educates such patients to a better diet which will not form further gall-stones.

Shiatsu should never be used for cancer because so stimulating is the massage to the flow of body fluids and energy that cancer cells can easily be spread from the tumour around the body. Apart from this there are no reasons why Shiatsu shouldn't be done in most people.

I have mentioned a first-aid application of Shiatsu already but there are others. Leg cramps can easily be cured by deep pressure between the roots of the big and second toes for ten to fifteen seconds. There is also a drowning point (between the anus and the genitals) which, when stimulated, causes the drowning person to exhale violently and so blow out the water. As an interesting historical note it's fascinating to think that students of the ancient martial arts centuries ago used to be trained in visual diagnosis. They would be able to tell a man's weak points at sight and then go for the respective acupuncture point to disable him. This has today been harnessed for more constructive purposes and hundreds of thousands of people throughout the western world are at last beginning to share in this ancient art that has proven so useful to the Japanese for more than thirty centuries.

Sound Therapy

Definition

The use of sound waves to heal.

Background

Sound waves can be a powerful force for good or bad but in sound therapy are used to help the body heal itself. Modern science has harnessed sound waves of very high frequency and employed them in the diagnostic tool known as the ultrasonic scanner which has now taken its place among the most useful of medical diagnostic aids. At the other end of the scale, extremely low frequency sound is said to be being explored by the military as a potential weapon which will act by conducting sound waves enormous distances through the earth's crust.

But in between these two are the vast numbers of sound wavelengths that immediately surround our audible sound range. We are all aware of the effects of noise upon our daily lives – at one end of the spectrum we are simply annoyed by it and at the other we may literally be driven mad by it. Studies have shown that people living around large international airports are more likely to have to go into a mental hospital than those living in quieter parts. Research has now proved conclusively that we 'hear' sounds while we are asleep and that they affect the quality of our sleep. People living near busy roads respond to noise (as shown by continuous night time brain-wave traces) and they are not as rested as when they sleep without noise around them. High levels of environmental noise at work, for example, can cause deafness if endured over a long period and most sound wavelengths have an effect on one part or another of our bodies. It is no accident that the screaming, hysterical masses at a pop concert behave the way they do – the powerful sound waves undoubtedly vibrate their internal organs. In fact it has been suggested that certain bass notes vibrate the pelvic organs of women and that this is why they find bass rhythmic music pleasant. Plants too it seems find music pleasant because they grow better when exposed to music than when exposed to random everyday noise!

Sound has a very basic significance to us all. In fact we may well find that the sound qualities of a person's voice might be significant in our liking or disliking him. Dr Hans Jenny developed an instrument called a 'tonoscope' which made it possible to visualize sound in three dimensions. Using the human voice as the source he was able to show, for example, that the letter O spoken into a microphone produced a perfectly spherical pattern on the tonoscope.

There are remarkable similarities in what constitutes basic and important sounds within cultures. In Matra Yoga there is a sound which is said to be the basis of everything, OM or AUM. The Hindu Mandykya Upanishad says, 'All that is, past, present and future – is truly OM. That which is beyond the triple conception of time is also OM.' Tibetans, Buddhists, Lamas, the Chinese, Japanese and Indonesians also have a similar interpretation of OM. Christians and Jews say AMEN and Muslims AMIN. When St John wrote in his Gospel, 'In the beginning was the word', he was probably emphasizing the ancient and widespread belief that the spoken word has far deeper significance than simply imparting information.

The Ancient Egyptians understood the relationship of form and substance to tone and Wachsmuth, a pupil of Rudolf Steiner (see page 93), developed very complex theories about the propagation of sound in relation to the very nature of Man and the universe that surrounds him. Healing prayers and indeed prayers of all kinds often rely on repetitive sounds having a fundamental effect on those praying. This is perhaps best seen in the mantras used in Ayurvedic medicine.

Sound therapy harnesses sound waves for healing purposes but uses as its basic principle the very facts that we have just been briefly considering – namely that each tissue in the body and every organ has its own 'vibrating' frequency which can be altered by the application of sound waves.

As we learn more about molecular structure and atomic physics we're realizing that every substance right down to its most fundamental sub-atomic particles is in a state of continuous vibration. A cell in the human body therefore is like a little battery – full of energy fields and 'vibrating' in a microscopic energy sense. The life processes going on in the cell emit this energy constantly in health but do so in a deranged way when the cell becomes diseased. The simplest and best known application of this principle in everyday medicine is the electrocardiogram. A series of electrodes placed on the skin over the heart and at places distant from it (the wrists and ankles) record the state of electrical 'vibrations' or frequencies generated by the heart. These can be examined on a TV-type screen or printed out on paper for posterity. When the heart muscle becomes damaged (for instance by a heart attack), the readings of the output are changed in such a characteristic way that doctors can tell simply by looking at the paper trace what is happening in the various parts of the heart and can pinpoint with considerable accuracy the part of the heart affected by disease. As the patient recovers, the ECG returns to normal as the electrical patterns themselves return to normal.

Sound therapists maintain that all of our organs and cells behave rather like the heart (if not quite as dramatically) and that all disease is manifest by a change in the fundamental frequency of the vibration or energy output of the body. This change can take place in a group of cells, a whole body organ or over the entire body. Sound therapy aims at bringing the vibrations back to normal.

Light has long been used for curative purposes and infra-red and ultra-violet lamps are well known both inside medicine and to the general public. These energy sources are simply generating vibrations of a different kind compared with the generators that sound therapists use. The end point is just the same though – the returning of the damaged or diseased tissue to its normal state.

How is it done?

Before discussing the practical details, let's just look at the background to sound therapy at the sound wave level. Waves are familiar to us all. Waves on the sea make us ill, waves in the air give us TV and radio. But they all have one thing in common – they compress the medium through which they are passing and then, a fraction of a second later, rarefy it. So a wave passes through a medium (water, air or body tissues, for example) by a series of compression and rarefaction waves. Our ears are sensitive only to a very small range of sound waves just as our eyes can only detect a small range of light frequencies.

Sound therapy involves the generation of sound waves by electronic devices. These waves are then delivered to the body by an applicator which is placed over the affected part needing treatment. The undesirable frequencies which are generated by the disease process are thus cancelled out and healing allowed to proceed.

The sound applicator is a simple hand-held instrument which delivers sounds from magnetic tapes which have been produced in the light of experience to deliver just the right wavelength for a particular tissue or organ. The applicator means that sound can be aimed and focused accurately rather than simply sitting the patient in a 'bath' of sound. A sound applicator isn't simply a vibrator as is used in massage – the sound frequency patterns delivered are complex and highly specific to the organ being treated.

When a person is having sound therapy he may or may not feel or hear the vibrations. Even if the patient does feel the applicator vibrating, he may well not feel the frequency which is the healing one and that is being 'heard' by the internal organs.

What is it used for?

Sound therapy is of greatest value (as far as we can say today anyway) in the treatment of rheumatoid arthritis, fibrositis, muscular conditions, fractures and bone disorders, strains and sprains. These areas have been the most obvious to treat with sound therapy because they are easily accessible to sound applicators but these are now also being used in treating internal disorders.

Sound therapists stress the importance of getting the diagnosis right before effecting a cure with sound. An arthritic condition that is really a manifestation of a psychological disorder can and will be improved with sound therapy but not for long unless the underlying disorder is treated properly too. About 80 per cent of all the cases seen by one leading sound therapist in the UK are of traumatic origin – even though the injury may have been sustained many years before the arthritis or other musculo-skeletal disease presents. This therapist also finds that patients about to undergo hip replacement operations fare a lot better after receiving pre-operative sound treatment. Patients pre-treated in this way heal much quicker and are up and about sooner than other patients. He maintains that sound therapy can do away with a lot of what physiotherapists do simply because it is quick, quiet, easy and needs no exertion on the patient's part.

Although rheumatoid arthritis can be helped by sound, according to Peter Guy Manners, a leading British sound therapy expert, if the joints are severely damaged, all he can hope for is an increase in joint mobility. However, to the chronic rheumatoid patient this can be a wonderful improvement. He also has good results with slipped discs and finds that sound, because it doesn't involve any manipulative treatment (which can be so painful for these patients), is very popular. The applicator is placed over the affected area for ten to fifteen minutes with the muscle and bone tapes running. This can relieve muscle spasm and so allow manipulation to be done if necessary. Classical lumbago also responds to this kind of treatment.

But sound therapy isn't just of use to the aged with degenerative diseases – it is used in babies and children too. Manners has used sound in children with muscle weakness and even cases of paralysis have responded, albeit over a long period.

The future

Sound therapy should have a bright future. It is a cheap, easily controllable therapy that deserves far greater research. The public and the medical world have seen what ultrasound can do in the treatment of soft tissue injuries and should be able to accept this supplementary medical therapy more readily than most. As long as care is taken to ensure that the healing waves for one organ or tissue don't cause disruption or damage to other tissues, sound therapy must be set for a secure future.

Yoga

Definition

Yoga (from the Sanscrit word for 'union' or 'oneness') is a personal self-help system of health care and spiritual development. It is not an alternative medicine as such but is very popular in the West and can be a positive benefit to the health of the practitioner if practised in accordance with the rules.

Background

Yoga is difficult to date as it has probably been practised in one form or another for thousands of years. Yoga positions have been found engraved on seals dating from 3000 BC. The great founders of yoga as we know it were working in India about 2,000 years ago and probably the distinguished yogi was an Indian sage, Patanjali, who wrote one of the major textbooks on the subject which remains a classic today. He described yoga as 'controlling the waves of the mind' – little did he know how close he was to the truth.

Yoga is a systematic approach to becoming 'one with life' and is a meditational discipline that encourages and helps Man to achieve his highest potential in life. Over the years the great yogic masters have slowly unravelled the problems involved with each of man's functions. These functions of the body were very carefully and systematically explored through a precise series of postures or *asanas* and it is these that make up what is known today as 'Hatha yoga'. Partly because yoga is a very ancient discipline, many different forms have grown up over the centuries, many centred on a guru (a dispeller of darkness). Mantra yoga is concerned mostly with the vibrations and radiations of life; Karma yoga is a kind of service in action and encourages service to others; Bhakti yoga's path is via devotion and love; Layakriya yoga uses the path of sexual relationships to achieve fulfilment but, as we've seen, Hatha yoga is the yoga mainly concerned with health through mastery of the body.

Over many years, the intricacies of breathing and posture have been studied so that easily reproducible movements and postures can be made to produce predictable effects on the body's function and so prevent or cure disease.

Because it was obvious that yoga actually changed basic bodily functions, scientists studied the changes in the laboratory and today there is a mass of experimental proof that yoga can have beneficial effects.

How is it done?

The postures of yoga range from sitting positions to movements aimed at toning the body and making it supple. Each posture has three main components – a bodily movement, a mental control process and a specific control of respiration. Great stress is put on correct breathing. Yogis maintain that breathing is the centre of our whole lives not only because it obviously gives us the oxygen we need to breathe but also because it vitalizes the autonomic nervous system. People who are tense, they maintain, breathe shallowly and in an irregular and uncontrolled way. Many yogis then start off by getting the subject breathing properly, using his diaphragm. Slow, controlled breathing calms the body and mind and so allows the practitioner to get deeper into a state of meditation. At this stage the body's life forces are, it is claimed, more in harmony than usual and any disordered systems of the body can thus be normalized.

Many yogis won't take on a new pupil unless he dedicates himself to self-discipline, cleanliness and a real desire to rid himself of the constraints of the western world. Some yogis insist on vegetarianism for their pupils. But these sorts of rigorous disciplines are unlikely to be adhered to by the average westerner who wants to use yoga as a pleasant and spiritually elevating pastime.

Does it work?

The answer is undoubtedly 'yes'. Yoga really is the high point of the various therapies involving mind over matter. Studies carried out all over the world have shown that there are provable physical benefits from practising yoga and the millions of practitioners world wide will attest to its efficacy. It was in the 1920s in Lonavala in India that the first laboratory to study yoga was set up and since then there have been thousands of studies, many of which are published in the learned medical and scientific literature.

Electromyographic studies, for example, show that people trained in yoga perform the *asanas* using far less muscular effort than do other fit, healthy people and that the practice of yoga makes people more flexible physically.

Manoeuvres known as the 'locks' involve controlling the diaphragm and the anal sphincter. In one type of abdominal lock the idea is to exhale completely and then make a mock inhalation. X-ray studies have shown that the diaphragm rises to a greater extent than during a normal expiration when this manoeuvre is performed; that the colon is raised (in its transverse portion) and, instead of sagging, may actually arch upwards. Such changes in intra-abdominal pressure also cause changes in the pressures within the internal abdominal organs and affect their functioning.

Other yoga manoeuvres enable the practitioner to perform feats of strength that are quite inexplicable in terms of his normal body power. One such demonstration by an Indian yogi of sixty-seven involved the 'breaking of a chain in two by winding it around the waist and extending it with the foot'. The chain, made of ⅜ inch iron bar gradually gave way under the pressure.

The circulatory system too can be greatly stimulated by yoga.

Certain postures, notably the so-called peacock posture, greatly increase the blood flow to certain abdominal organs such as the pancreas. Some important postures involve standing on the head or shoulders so that the body is upside down. Blood is thus pooled in the head and neck by simple gravity and especially benefits the pituitary gland, the main control centre of the endocrine system. By careful pressure of the chin in a particular part of the neck, the blood flow to the thyroid gland can be modified and the actual temperature of the gland itself rises as its blood flow is enhanced. Swami Rama, a particularly gifted yogi, can so selectively alter the bloodflow to various parts of his body that studies using thermistors have demonstrated a 10°C temperature difference between two points on one of his hands. This opens up considerable possibilities in the treatment of certain very vascular cancers, as their growth could possibly be arrested or slowed if their blood flow could be kept low. Yogis can alter their heart rates too and some expert practitioners have such control that they can actually stop their hearts altogether. Blood pressure can also be altered at will with practice and an article in the *British Medical Journal* of 1976 went so far as to claim that yoga and meditation might become a serious form of treatment for hypertension within a few years. Using biofeedback equipment, Dr Patel, a general practitioner working in suburban London, teaches her patients to use yoga relaxation to lower their blood pressures. Groups of patients using yoga biofeedback training consistently had lower blood pressures than control patients.

Breathing too is altered considerably by yoga. Yogis can reduce their breathing rate to one or two breaths per minute (the normal is about twenty) or raise it to 120 per minute at will.

But it's the changes in brain wave rhythms that are particularly interesting because, simply by controlled breathing, yogis can induce alpha rhythms at will and produce altered states of mind. The brain wave rhythms also change during meditation and other types of wave can be induced at will. Swami Rama, for example, could induce theta waves 75 per cent of the time. These waves are usually only seen at the transition between the waking and sleeping states but have also been shown to be associated with periods of high creativity.

What of the future?

The trouble with studying and practising yoga is that it originates from an entirely alien culture to ours and so almost needs translating into concepts that a western mind can grasp. Much of it is highly philosophical and problems arise with poor translations from Bengali, Sanscrit or Prakrit.

However, positive health benefits can be achieved over long periods of yoga, especially if it is practised under controlled conditions or as a group activity and under the watchful eye of an expert. Because so many very real physiological changes can be induced, it is essential to be sure that do-it-yourself efforts don't harm instead of help.

Yoga is no panacea but most people find they get a feeling of improved mental well-being after a couple of months of regular practice. In my opinion, the other 'medical' benefits require much more devotion and serious training than all but the keenest western practitioner is likely to undertake. In good hands and combined with biofeedback training it can be useful in specific diseases such as hypertension but even this is highly unlikely to become a major therapeutic tool.

Index